Zen and the Art of Cooking Beer-Can Chicken

Welcome to the new Zen infused world of cuckoo culinary delight!

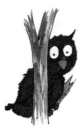

Red Owl Publications presents the Definitive Guide to Cooking Infusion Style Beer-Can Chicken!

Get ready to make your grilling, roasting or baking poultry easier, tastier, goofier and more outrageous!

By
Cary Black

Illustrated By
Donald Black

1st edition published under the title:

Zen Chicken and the Art of Continuous Infusion © 2004

2nd edition entitled:

Zen and the Art of Cooking Beer-Can Chicken: The Definitive Guide

Third printing contains minor editorial changes.

ISBN 0-9754279-1-1

12345678910

Book design: Cary Black
Illustrations: Donald Black
Cover Design: Gerry Mercieca, Eclipse Graphic Design, Midland, MI

Published by Red Owl Publications, L.L.C
P.O. Box 446
Freeland, MI 48623

www.redowlpublications.com

Printed by Signature Book Printing, Gaithersburg, MD, USA

First printing, October, 2005
Second printing, June, 2006
Third printing: November, 2007

Acknowledgments

Many people contributed to the efforts at creating this cookbook. To my family and all those friends who in some way had tokens of advice, words of support and encouragement. Great thanks go to my father, Don Black, who enthusiastically churned out chicken cartoons by the dozens and helped keep this work fun and light spirited. Special thanks go out to my family who put up with my many hours of absence as I labored in front of a computer.

Further acknowledgments are extended to Brenda Buehneman of Sigourney, Iowa and my mother, Gretchen George for their contributions of amazing dessert recipes. Thanks also to Angi Dodge for her marketing and editorial contributions to the chicken and turkey recipes. Thanks to my colleagues in the No Regrets rock and roll band. Thanks go out to Phil Nanzetta of Signature Book Printing for his help in tying the loose ends together. Thanks also go out to my friends and colleagues at Duro-Last for their support. Thanks also to Chad Koralik of Chadwood Graphic Designs for his internet support. Thanks also to Rick Kazdan who taught me much about the importance of communication in the course of doing business.

Special thanks to Tom Simon, Sean Black (you are the best), Todd Fritz, Al Janni, Gerry Mercieca, Steve Vinson, Kimmy Dunn, Victor Sapirstein, Ruis Peres, Mark Ouellette, and Tom Hollingsworth. Thank you all.

This book is dedicated to all those people whose lives were changed by the hurricanes Katrina and Rita. It is further dedicated to those men and women who are putting their lives on the line for our great country… it is my thoughts and prayers that you all find your way home whole and at peace.

This book is also dedicated to the loving memory of my beautiful step-mother Danielle. May your heavenly journey, be full of beauty and grace.

I wish you all peace and pray for harmony and joy in all your lives.

Cary

"What wonders the Universe presents to us in our lives, in our fortunes, and our mutual perspectives…is forever challenged and made whole through thoughtful perceptions and philosophical evolution from friends, colleagues and loved ones…I wish you all peace, my friends!! May we all view the world through clear eyes and with love in our hearts!"

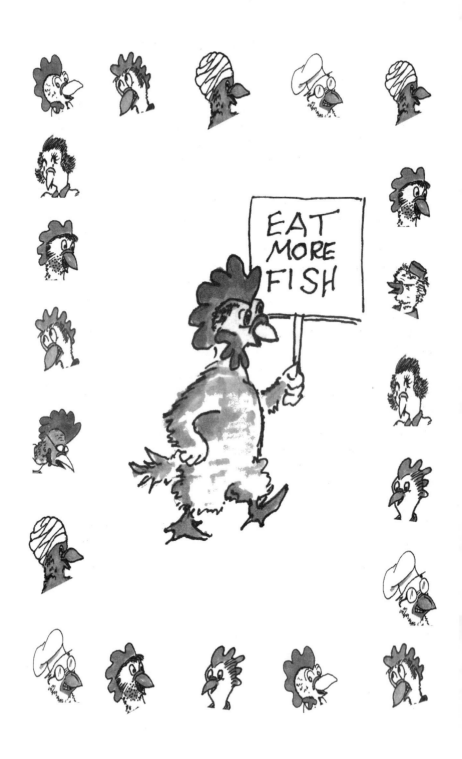

Table of Contents

Brining

Injecting

Zen Chicken Recipes (continued)

Assorted Appetizers and Sides

Assorted Appetizers and Sides
(continued)

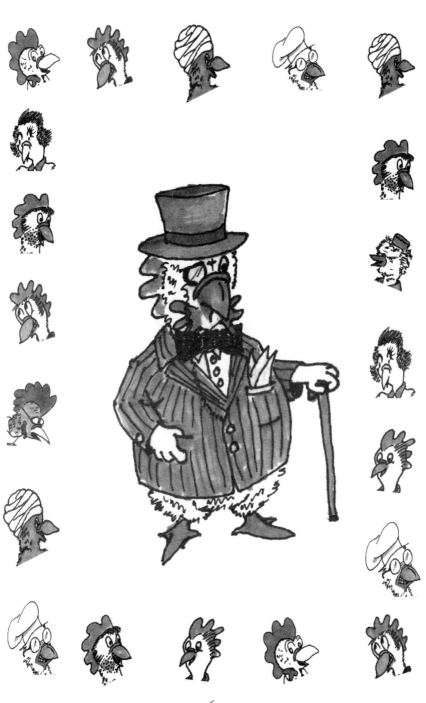

Cooking Beer-Can Chicken

Author's Preface

Zen Chicken and the Art of Continuous Infusion! Now here is an idea with some interesting connotations.

When I think of Zen, or at least applying the principles of Zen to an endeavor, I think of simplicity, elegance, creativity and balance. The recipes in this cookbook are designed to be simple, fun and great tasting. This cookbook was written such that you, dear reader, can input your own creative culinary impulses as you explore this unique approach to cooking chicken.

The concept of continuous infusion describes a process of cooking where moist vapor is circulated through the food while cooking.

It all started with the concept of "Beer-can" chicken and was followed by the invention of many fine infusion cookers designed to emulate the beer-can chicken cooking experience.

The Beginning

The story begins with a creatively inclined individual who had grown tired of the same old mundane chow. This individual enjoyed fresh poultry and decided to try something new and different.

Being a connoisseur of fine beer, this person thought, "Why not flavor this bird with a bit of brew?" This individual then cracked a can of his favorite brew and stuffed it up into a whole chicken found sleeping in the icebox.

A bit of garlic powder, a dash of salt and a smattering of pepper were rubbed over the outside of the bird and onto the grill it went.

As the temperature increased, the beer inside of the can began to boil. The steam, laden with the essence of hops and malt vapor, exited from the top of the can and began to cook the bird from the inside out.

After about an hour and a half, the bird emerged. The rub on the outside had incorporated into the crisp skin, locking in the bird juices. The meat under the skin was butter-knife tender and gently flavored with the essence of hops.

The Inventions

Years later, creative entrepreneurs inspired by the simplicity and great taste of beer-can chicken began to invent infusion cookers to make the process simpler and better. This cookbook attests to three of the best chicken infusion cookers available today. Each of the cookers listed in this cookbook is of excellent quality, relatively inexpensive and will provide an awesome "beer-can" Zen chicken experience.

The Cookbook

In June of 2003, I had the privilege of working with Tom Simon the inventor of the Poultry Pal® through our respective place of employment. I had been hired as a contract technical writer and Tom was one of my key resources for the assignment. The timing of our meeting could not have been better, as Tom was in the initial phases of developing and patenting the Poultry Pal® infusion cooker.

Tom invited me to write some "tongue-in-cheek", humorous recipes for the initial pamphlet to be included with the product.

The list of recipes grew. The humor and fun inherent in the writing of this material took on a life of its own and the project ultimately became this cookbook. As the list of recipes grew (and following the humorous approach), I enlisted the aid of my father, Don Black, to draw cartoons representing the humorous aspect of the recipes.

This cookbook was been designed as a companion reference tool for beer-can chicken cooking using an array of the finest infusion cookers on the market.

I have included the directions for using a beer-can to cook your poultry…but only do so with the understanding that you will invest in one of the fine products supported by this cookbook. You see, most beer-cans are coated in inks that are non food-grade. Much ink used in beer-cans may have toxic effects when exposed to the types of temperatures typically used for cooking. Further, beer-cans are made from aluminum. At typical cooking temperatures, aluminum vapors will transfer from the can to the meat to unacceptable levels for human consumption.

It is highly recommended that to avoid ingesting these toxins, you should purchase one of the fine products designed to emulate and improve the beer-can chicken experience. All of the inexpensive products represented within this book will safely offer up simple and delicious meals. A hint of the unusual, a bit of Zen creativity and amazingly great food all await you as you venture onto the path of "beer-can" continuous infusion cooking.

The infusion cooking process drains away unhealthy fat, as flavor-rich moistness imparts subtle flavors to the bird.

The cooking process incorporates a continuous infusion of flavor vapor up the flavor tower, with fats draining away from the chicken.

The design of these infusion cookers is such that vegetables can also be cooked with the bird. They can be lined up around the base of the chicken or added to the liquid libation in the flavor base for extra flavor and tenderness.

A three to six lb. whole chicken will feed four to six people. The prep time is minimal and the clean up is a breeze. Have fun! Save money! And please even the most discerning palates. Welcome to a brave, new and definitely Zen-ish world of culinary creation!

I have included recipes for great rubs, sauces, brines, injectables, accompaniments and desserts to go with the fine poultry cooked with the continuous infusion cookers.

Please sit back, enjoy the read, eat well and smile a lot, bless your children and friends, be at peace, be creative and indulge to your heart's content!

Cary Black, October, 2005

Visit our website at:
www.redowlpublications.com

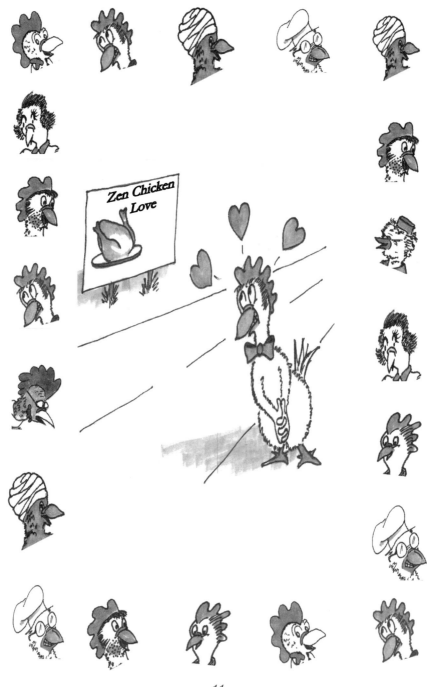

Zen and the Art of...

*An expression of
heavenly bliss can be found
simply with the casual
enjoyment of a
continuously infused
chicken.*

The Poultry Pal® Infusion Cooker

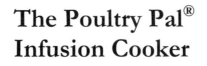

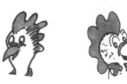
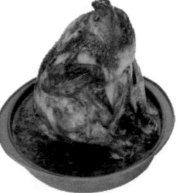

The Poultry Pal®

Tom Simon of Bay City, Michigan, had always enjoyed beer-can chicken. One day while cleaning out his wife's pantry, he discovered a miniature bundt cake pan. Being adventurous and having a desire for beer-can chicken for supper, he took the bundt cake pan out to the shed and drilled some holes in the tower and the base. Placing it over an old pie pan filled with beer and using a simple barbecue rub, he cooked his chicken. The family was quite impressed and at that particular supper, the Poultry Pal® Cooker was born.

Poultry Pal® Cooker, one of my favorites, represents a true continuous infusion cooking process. The drippings from the bird find their way back to the flavor base for a continuous infusion of flavor during cooking.

Tom patented the design and began producing the cooker. The rest is history. Without Tom and the Poultry Pal®, this book would not have been possible.

The Poultry Pal® continues to sell on the Home Shopping Network while Poultry Pal, LLC's network of distribution continues to grow in leaps and bounds.

In addition to the cooker, Poultry Pal carries a fine line of spices and accessories that accompany the infusion cooker.

Poultry Pal® products can be purchased on the Internet at:

www.redowlpublications.com

Cluck-n-Stuff
Beer Butt
Chicken Heads

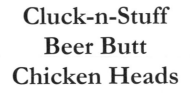

Cluck-n-Stuff Beer Butt Chicken Heads

Once upon a time at an afternoon barbeque in Boise, Idaho, some creative folks with overactive imaginations were grilling some beer-can chicken. While enjoying the company of friends and sipping their cold frosty beers, they would periodically check the chicken for doneness. After lifting the grill lid for the third time they decided that there is something horribly wrong with the chicken. No, it wasn't the way the chicken was cooking; it was the way the chicken was looking. There it was just sitting there without a head; it was at that point they had light bulb moment......"This chicken needs a head!"

They started dressing up a potato with eyes, ears, nose, and a tin foil hat. Kind of like an edible Mr. Potato head. They thought there might be something to the chicken head phenomena, and thus started playing with clay to see what might be possible. Working with Anthony Bulone, who is a master mold maker and the designer of the original Barbie Doll, they came up with some prototype molds. Soon they were cranking out Beer-Butt Chicken heads from their living room."

Since developing the Beer Butt Chicken Heads and forming the company Cluck-n-Stuff, Dan and Robyn Asimus have taken the product on the road to the National Fiery Foods and BBQ Show in Albuquerque, NM. The ceramic heads were a huge success. The heads won several awards. Many shows later, a booming website, multiple television appearances and a marketing collaboration with Red Owl Publications and Poultry Pal have taken Cluck-n-Stuff to new levels of business.

The ceramic heads fit perfectly into the neck of your beer-can chicken or turkey. They give a new perspective to the culinary concept of "presentation", and help keep the infused moisture inside the bird where it belongs.

www.redowlpublications.com

The Chickāno Porcelain Infusion Cooker

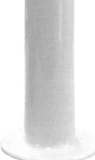

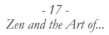

The Chickāno
Porcelain Infusion Cooker

Mary Lazier and Mark Tichenor formed Little Red Hen's Kitchen Garden in 1995 as a home based business to produce and market their pottery. Located in Mansfield, Ontario, Canada, Little Red Hen's Kitchen Garden supplies a delightful array of functional and artistic pottery products. Mary and Mark both started out as technical professionals but opted out to a simpler, more satisfying lifestyle as artisans and entrepreneurs.

The Chickāno started out with their daughter Sara, requesting they make her a pottery chicken cooker for making "beer-can" chicken. She wanted to try "beer-can" chicken, but didn't like the idea of putting a plastic lined, painted aluminum beer-can inside her food to cook it.

The first design worked well and they were amazed at the succulent flavor it gave the chicken. However, the prototype was a bit too heavy to ship at a reasonable price. The second design worked well in the oven, but tended to break on the grill. Mark set out to torture-test the prototype product on the grill. After breaking a half dozen cookers, it became obvious that the base (which was in full contact with the metal pan) was heating much too fast, while the cylinder filled with beer remained cool. Crack!

To remedy the situation, Mark tried adding a small foot-ring as part of the porcelain body to achieve the separation from the cooking pan. It worked like a charm with no more cracking.

You can order the Chickāno and many other fine products at:

www.redowlpublications.com

Jazz on Continuous Infusion

➤ The infusion cookers were designed and patented to create simple and versatile ways to cook chicken and other small bird-like creatures.

➤ The flavor tower was designed to conveniently accommodate an array of vegetables or giblets around the base of the chicken to minimize or eliminate the need for other pans and pots while cooking.

➤ The flavor base was designed to also accommodate vegetables and giblets to baste and cook within the liquid flavor medium if desired.

➤ As the temperature rises, the liquid flavor essence begins to boil, releasing subtle flavor vapors, which rise up through the flavor tower and permeate the chicken from the inside.

➤ As the bird cooks, fats and juices run down to the base of the flavor tower and drain into the flavor base. A continuous infusion of flavor vapor and steam is established, cooking the bird from the inside out and imparting moisture and subtle flavor into the meat. The draining of the fat into the flavor base engenders a much healthier meal, significantly reduced in fat but enhanced in flavor.

➤ A good rub on the outside of the bird helps lock the flavor inside and provides for a crispy and tasty outer surface.

The Incredible Invisible Bird on an Infusion Cooker

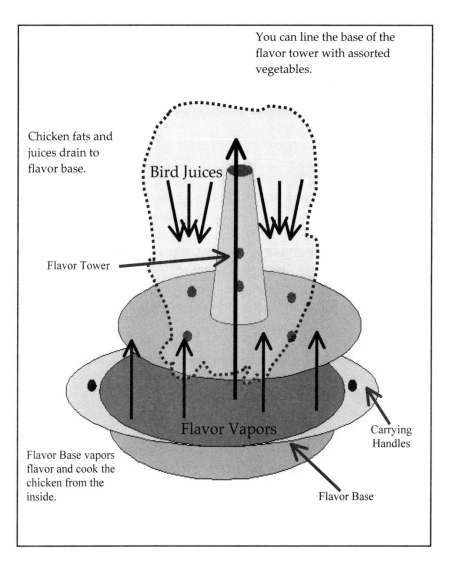

You can line the base of the flavor tower with assorted vegetables.

Chicken fats and juices drain to flavor base.

Bird Juices

Flavor Tower

Flavor Vapors

Carrying Handles

Flavor Base vapors flavor and cook the chicken from the inside.

Flavor Base

Safety First

➢ Prior to use, thoroughly wash the cooker with detergent. A clean Poultry Pal® makes for a far superior chicken.

➢ As with all poultry products, care should be taken in handling the raw meat. Thoroughly wash all raw poultry products, cooking devices and utensils before and after preparation.

➢ The cooker is hot when cooking is complete. The liquid in the flavor base will be boiling. Always use hot pads or oven mitts when handling your cooker during and after cooking.

➢ Do not store raw or cooked poultry products with other foodstuffs.

➢ Check that the bird is completely cooked. The drippings should be clear and the leg quarters should move freely in their joints. If desired, a meat thermometer can be inserted into the thigh away from the bone. The temperature should be about 180°.

➢ Since the preparation of continuous infusion recipes often involves the use of liquids containing alcohol, both in the actual cooking and in the socialization intrinsic to the process, it is important to drink responsibly!

➢ If you decide to try pure high alcohol content liquors as your flavor liquid, remember that alcohol is flammable. It is recommended to dilute pure spirits with at least 50% water prior to cooking to prevent flame-ups during cooking.

The Basics

We've included some tried and true recipes that you will find exciting and easy. Use ours or make your own. Experiment, create and ponder the meaning of life within a tasty tender bird...

Basic Bird Preparation:

➤ Remove the giblets and neck.

➤ Remove and discard the fat just inside of the body.

➤ Clean the bird with warm water inside and out.

➤ Pour just a bit of lemon or lime juice inside the bird and shake to drain.

➤ Dry thoroughly with a clean cloth or paper towels.

➤ Season bird inside and out.

➤ Slide bird onto the flavor tower with its legs pointing down.

➤ Brush outside of bird with some oil... Be creative! Vegetable oil, olive oil, peanut oil or sesame oil are all fair game.

➤ Pour 12 to 15 oz. of your liquid flavor substance into the flavor base.

➤ Place the flavor tower, with bird in place, onto flavor base and cook the little buzzard!

➤ All temperatures in this book are reported in degrees F.

Continuous Infusion Tips and Toodles

➤ Wash the cooker with mild dish detergent before using.

➤ For yuks, try throwing a handful of vegetables around the chicken at the base of the flavor tower.

➤ You can zest up the liquid libation in the flavor base by throwing onions, garlic or peppers into the flavor base. Try cooking the giblets in the flavor base for some extra treats.

➤ When using the Poultry Pal®, do not overfill the flavor base. Use only 12 to 15 oz. of liquid (or 8 oz. when preparing a 10-14 lb. turkey). As the bird cooks, liquid and fat will return to the flavor base. For the Vertical Chicken Roaster and the Chickāno, fill the flavor towers until they are nearly full. Use a supporting casserole or pie dish under the Chickāno to catch the drippings.

➤ Carefully remove the bird from the tower before carving.

➤ Dry rubs will result in a crispier and more flavorful skin. Apply to both the outside and inside of the bird.

➤ Barbecue Sauce results in a moist, tender skin. Because of the sugar content of most Barbecue Sauces, it is recommended to baste bird after 40 minutes or so of cooking to avoid burning.

➤ Rotating the infusion cooker halfway through cooking will aid in even browning.

➤ To avoid spilling the hot liquid, carefully remove the cooker from the grill or oven using hot pads or oven mitts. Dispose of the liquid properly.

➤ If you are grilling, throw some mesquite or hickory wood chips into the grill for additional flavor. Try soaking the chips in water overnight, wrapping them up in an aluminum foil pouch and perforating the pouch. Such an approach makes for easy disposal after cooking.

Generic Cooking Directions

Gas Grills

➤ Place the chicken cooker with bird on the side of your grill with the lowest heat setting.

➤ Turn the other burner up to medium-high, ideally to 350°.

➤ Add flavor wood chips, if desired. Close lid.

➤ If your grill tends to burn hot, you can put an aluminum foil tent over the bird to assure desired skin texture. Remove in the last 15 minutes of cooking.

➤ Cook approximately 1¼ to 1½ hours or until drippings run clear and leg quarters move easily in their joints.

➤ If using a highly sugared basting sauce or coating, cook at 325°. for 1½ to 2 hours or until done.

➤ The inner thigh meat should be about 175 to 180°.

➤ Remove from heat and let stand for five minutes.

➤ Carefully remove bird from tower before carving.

Charcoal Grill

➤ Using _the indirect cooking method_, rake glowing coals into equal piles at opposite ends of the grill. Add flavor wood chips, if desired.

➤ Place the chicken cooker holding the bird in the center of the grill between piles of coals.

➤ If your grill tends to burn hot, you can put an aluminum foil tent over the bird to assure desired skin texture. Remove in the last 15 minutes of cooking.

➤ Cook approximately 1¼ to 1½ hours or until drippings run clear and leg quarters move easily in their joints.

➤ If using a highly sugared basting sauce or coating, cook at 325° for 1½ to 2 hours or until done.

➤ The inner thigh meat should be about 175 to 180°.

➤ Remove from heat and let stand for five minutes.

➤ Carefully remove bird from tower before carving.

Oven Method

➤ Pre-heat oven to 350°.

➤ Place the chicken cooker holding the bird on lowest rack. The bird should not touch top of oven.

➤ If desired, some foil or a baking sheet can be used to protect oven bottom; although, with care in handling, this is probably not necessary.

➤ Cook approximately 1¼ to 1½ hours or until drippings run clear and leg quarters move easily in their joints.

➤ If using a highly sugared basting sauce or coating, cook at 325° for 1½ to 2 hours or until done.

➤ The inner thigh meat should be about 175 to 180° F.

➤ Remove from heat and let stand for five minutes.

➤ Carefully remove bird from tower before carving.

Standard Beer-can Chicken Cooking

For those of you chicken connoisseurs who have not yet acquired an infusion cooker and desire to explore the world of beer-can chicken, the following instructions will help you in your cause. A fine tasty bird can be cooked using the beer-can method; however, this method loses the continuous infusion process elements provided by the infusion cookers. The beer-can method can be done using an oven or grill following the cooking directions cited on pages 23 through 26. Try the beer-can approach and if you like the results, buy an infusion cooker and enter the wonderful world of Zen and the Art of Cooking Beer-Can Chicken.

Note that many beer-cans have polymeric linings and non-food rated inks. Aluminum is also toxic. It is highly recommended that one use the fine infusion cooker included in this cookbook for the best and healthiest "beer-can" chicken.

Directions

➢ Wash the can with soapy water and rinse well.

➢ Open the can and discard about ¼ of the contents.

➢ Using a can opener or a small screwdriver, poke more holes in the top of the can, both on the top and at various points below the top, and on the sides of the can. This will allow for improved steam distribution during the cooking process.

➢ It is recommended to use a rectangular baking pan or cookie sheet to catch the drippings during cooking.

➢ Once the chicken has been cleaned and spiced with your favorite rub, insert the can into the chicken and carefully place in the pan, using the legs to complete a tripod configuration with the can.

➢ Cook as previously described on pages 23 through 26.

➢ Visit any of the websites listed in this book to order an infusion cooker.

Basic Rubs and Marinades

The dry rub applied to the outside of the bird is a great way to enhance and embellish the flavor and appearance of the critter being cooked. I have included a list of rubs that have proved tasty and provocative. Try some of these or create your own! Again, creativity is the live-wire...play with what you like...experiment, stand on your head and cluck like a chicken...or sing to the Universe for divine Zen rub inspiration.

Furthermore, I have included some tried and true marinades for those with a little more time to prepare the ultimate in chicken culinary concoctions.

Enjoy, embellish, create and enjoy. Observe the intensity and delight your eaters will exhibit while savoring the wonders of a tasty bird dancing upon and titillating their palates.

Basic Rubs

Uncle Tom's Basic Rub

➢ ¼ c. Kosher or Sea Salt
➢ ¼ c. brown sugar
➢ ¼ c. sweet or hot paprika
➢ ground pepper to taste

Mix the ingredients together in a bowl using your fingers. Store in an airtight container, away from heat. Use vegetable or olive oil on the chicken so the rub adheres well to the bird.

Cajun Cuckoo Rub

- ➢ ¼ c. Kosher or Sea Salt
- ➢ ¼ c. ground cayenne pepper
- ➢ ¼ c. brown sugar
- ➢ ¼ c. ground cumin
- ➢ ¼ c. garlic powder
- ➢ ground pepper to taste

Mix the ingredients together in a bowl using your fingers. Store in an airtight container, away from heat. Use vegetable or olive oil on the chicken so the rub adheres well to the bird.

Cacciatore Bliss

- ➢ ¼ c. Kosher or Sea Salt
- ➢ ¼ c. ground rosemary
- ➢ ¼ c. ground oregano
- ➢ ¼ c. garlic powder
- ➢ ground pepper to taste

Mix the ingredients together in a bowl using your fingers. Store in an airtight container, away from heat. Use a mixture of red wine and olive oil on the chicken so the rub adheres well to the bird.

European Herbal Rub

➢ ½ c. Kosher or Sea Salt
➢ ½ c. ground rosemary
➢ ½ c. ground oregano
➢ ¼ c. garlic powder
➢ ½ c. basil
➢ ½ c. tarragon
➢ ½ c. thyme
➢ ground pepper to taste

Mix the ingredients together in a bowl using your fingers. Store in an airtight container, away from heat. Use a mixture of wine and olive oil or Italian salad dressing on the chicken so the rub adheres well to the bird.

Madness à la Mexico

➢ ¼ c. Kosher or Sea Salt
➢ ¼ c. cilantro
➢ ¼ c. chili powder
➢ ¼ c. garlic powder
➢ ¼ c. ground cayenne pepper
➢ ¼ c. ground cumin

Mix the ingredients together in a bowl using your fingers. Store in an airtight container, away from heat. Use a mixture of salsa and olive oil on the chicken so the rub adheres well to the bird.

Beijing Bistro Rub

- ¼ c. Kosher or Sea Salt
- ¼ c. chili powder
- ¼ c. dried sesame seeds
- ¼ c. brown sugar
- ¼ c. garlic powder
- ¼ c. celery powder

Mix the ingredients together in a bowl using your fingers. Store in an airtight container, away from heat. Use a mixture of sugar, peanut oil and soy sauce on the chicken so the rub adheres well to the bird.

Cinnamon Delight Rub

- ¼ c. Kosher or Sea Salt
- ¼ c. ground cinnamon
- ¼ c. brown sugar
- ¼ c. garlic powder
- ¼ c. ground black pepper

Mix the ingredients together in a bowl using your fingers. Store in an airtight container, away from heat. Apply olive oil liberally over the chicken. Apply the rub to the bird. Cook and enjoy.

Marinades and Sauces

A good marinade strongly influences the flavor of your chicken. Create your own or try some of the following. It is best to make enough marinade in a bowl or container large enough to completely immerse your delectable bird. Cover and refrigerate for a while...Bon Appétit!

Soak that bird for a while, sit back, enjoy, smile at your friends and loved ones, crack a brew or some fine wine and get that bird a'roastin' with the Zen and Harmony of continuous infusion, hoppy-essences and magnanimous musings.

All Season Buffalo Marinade

➢ 2 c. chili sauce
➢ 2 c. red wine vinegar
➢ 2 c. dry red wine
➢ 1½ Tbs. fresh ground horseradish
➢ ¼ c. ground cayenne pepper
➢ ¼ c. garlic powder
➢ ground pepper to taste

Mix all the ingredients. Immerse your bird in the marinade. Marinate for an hour or so. Dance with the zest of the rare Buffalo Bird!

South Pacific Floating Chicken

- ➤ 2 c. orange juice
- ➤ ½ c. honey
- ➤ 2 c. soy or teriyaki sauce
- ➤ 2 c. sake or dry white wine
- ➤ 1½ Tbs. fresh ground horseradish
- ➤ ¼ c. garlic powder
- ➤ ¼ c. pepper to taste
- ➤ ¼ c. dried sesame seeds
- ➤ 1 whole lime sectioned into eighths

Mix all the ingredients. Immerse your bird in the marinade. Marinate overnight in the refrigerator. Imagine sitting on the beach listening to the surf in the warm equatorial sun. Soaking up the rays and sippin' somethin' cool…

Burgundy Chicken Marinade

- ➤ 3 c. Burgundy
- ➤ 2 c. white tarragon vinegar
- ➤ 1 c. virgin olive oil
- ➤ ¼ c. garlic powder
- ➤ ¼ c. fine chopped onion
- ➤ ¼ c. pepper to taste

Mix all the ingredients. Immerse your bird in the marinade. Marinate overnight in the refrigerator. Images of the French countryside, with warm breezes blowing through red, grape-laden vines, will come unbidden as your palate gets a taste of this evocative concoction.

Roma La Pesto

➢ 2 c. olive oil
➢ 3 c. Chianti or dry red wine
➢ 2 c. basil
➢ 1 c. vinegar
➢ ½ c. garlic powder
➢ ¼ c. pepper to taste
➢ ¼ c. dried oregano
➢ ¼ c. dried rosemary

Mix all the ingredients. Immerse your bird into the marinade. Marinate for several hours in the refrigerator. The sweet essence of basil and garlic will flavor this bird. You can almost hear the splashing of the oars moving up and down the Viennese canals. Unfettered, free and emboldened with Old World flavor. Salut!

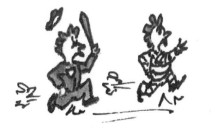
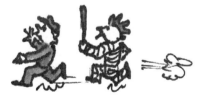

Mole Sauce

- ➢ 2 Tbs. butter
- ➢ 1 medium onion, finely grated
- ➢ 2 tsp. garlic powder
- ➢ 1 bay leaf
- ➢ ½ tsp. black pepper
- ➢ ½ tsp. ground cloves
- ➢ 1 c. tomato sauce
- ➢ 1 c. chicken broth
- ➢ ½ can finely chopped canned Chipotle peppers.
- ➢ 2 tsp. of Adobo sauce from Chipotle peppers
- ➢ ¼ tsp. anise seed
- ➢ ½ tsp. ground cinnamon
- ➢ ½ tsp. ground cumin
- ➢ 1 tsp. white sugar
- ➢ 2 Tbs. ground red chili pepper
- ➢ 2 oz. grated Mexican chocolate

Combine Mole sauce ingredients in a microwave safe container, cover and microwave on low to medium for five minutes. Stir and continue to heat as necessary to blend and liquefy the sauce. Let stand.

A fine mole works wonders with chicken. Try it with the Très Amigos chicken (page 58). Spice up your bird and sing a Mexican drinking song!

Note: You can purchase a small can (approx. 7 oz.) of Chipotle peppers in Adobo sauce in the Mexican food section of your grocer.

Caribbean Jerk Glaze

- 4 oz. habanero pepper sauce
- 1 c. orange marmalade
- ½ c. lime juice
- ½ c. grated coconut
- ½ c. dark brown sugar
- ¼ c. rum
- ¼ c. grated orange peel

Combine marmalade, orange peel, coconut, brown sugar, a splash of rum, lime juice and habanero pepper sauce (to taste). Stir well to assure a smooth consistency, cover and set aside. The mixture will store well in refrigerator for a month. Makes about 2½ cups. Resisting the urge to Tango while preparing this delightful delectable is advised.

Gravy à la Normandy

- 12 oz. of the liquid flavor drippings from the cooked Chicken Normandy bird (page 102).
- ½ c. whipping cream
- ¼ c. cornstarch

Add the liquid flavor drippings from the cooked Chicken Normandy (page 102), whipped cream and cornstarch to a saucepan and gently bring to a boil for 1 minute. Stir until thick and smooth.

A sip of a fine Chardonnay, the warm sun and vineyard fragrances wafting over the elegance of the French countryside comforts the soul... Trés Bonne!

Peking Peanut Sauce

- ➤ ½ c. teriyaki sauce
- ➤ ½ c. peanut butter
- ➤ 2 Tbs. peanut oil
- ➤ 1 Tbs. sugar
- ➤ 1 Tbs. powdered ginger
- ➤ 1 Tbs. garlic powder
- ➤ 1 tsp. Kosher or Sea Salt
- ➤ ½ tsp. powdered red pepper

Combine the teriyaki sauce, peanut oil, peanut butter, sugar and spices and mix until smooth. If necessary, add more teriyaki sauce until mixture is of desired consistency. Makes about 1½ cups.

A particularly fun and tasty recipe to enjoy while meditating upon a visit to the Great Wall or contemplating the serenity of a Shaolin temple.

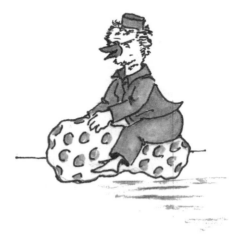

Brining and Injecting

No cookbook covering Zen and the Art of Beer-Can chicken cooking would be complete without a section on brining and injecting. The brining and injecting techniques represent alternative pre-treatments for enhancing the infusion cooking approach thus adding to your creative options.

Try some of the brines and injection recipes included within this book. Though optional, using these techniques can give you creative options thoroughly enhancing the flavor versatility of the infusion style of cooking.

Brine That Bird

The brining of meats was one of the first types of preservation ever practiced. The key to brining is the use of salt, which has from time immemorial been used to preserve meats prior to the days of refrigeration.

The practice of brining probably started with the Jewish practice of treating meat called "koshering". In this practice, meat was placed in containers and treated with Kosher salt. In koshering, the objective was to draw all of the blood out of the meat.

Indeed the galleys of the ancient mariners such as Christopher Columbus and Ferdinand Magellan were well stocked with brined meats for consumption over long months at sea.

In brining, the salt acts through processes of osmosis and diffusion. The brining process forces water into the proteins of the muscle tissues. This additional moisture causes the proteins of the meat to swell as they absorb more water. The additional moisture in the proteins allows for more moisture retention during cooking. With proper cooking, the result is meat with enhanced flavor and moisture. Spices added to the brine are also carried deep into the meat allowing creative flavor enhancements.

Because of the extra moisture in the meat tissues, brined birds take less time to cook as the additional moisture helps cook the meat fibers from within. Cooking times can be reduced up to 25 %. Care should be taken when cooking brined birds. The reduction in cooking time will depend on the length of time the bird soaked in the brine. Use a meat thermometer to assure the inner thigh meat is at 175° to 180° and to guarantee your bird is fully cooked.

It is recommended that for the 3 to 6 lb. birds, brine only for 4 to 6 hours. For larger poultry such as a 10 to 14 lb. turkey, brining for 10 to 16 hours is sufficient.

Brining Tips and Toodles

➢ Always brine in a refrigerator to assure minimal bacteria formation during the brining process.

➢ To determine how much brine to make, use a plastic container that has sufficient volume to completely immerse your bird. Measure the amount of water required and mix your brine to the appropriate concentration, as discussed below.

➢ Make sure that the whole bird is immersed in the brining solution. You can use a plate to weigh down the bird to assure complete coverage.

➢ When brining is complete, rinse the bird well and discard the brine. Cook your brined buzzard immediately.

➢ The salty flavor of the brine is offset and mellowed by using some kind of sweetening agent such as sugar, honey, maple syrup etc.

➢ When brining for the first time, use shorter brining times to avoid making your culinary creation too salty.

➢ If you have no room in your refrigerator, place your bird in a clean trash bag, pour in your brine assuring full immersion, seal and store in an ice filled cooler.

The Basic Bird Brine

Once you have determined how much brine is required to fully immerse your bird, use the following brine recipe:

> ➤ 1 gallon water
> ➤ 1¼ c. Kosher or Sea salt (or ¾ c. table salt)
> ➤ ¾ c. sugar (or ¾ c brown sugar)
> ➤ ¼ c. olive oil (optional)
> ➤ 1 Tbs. black pepper

Prepping Directions:

➤ Bring 1 quart of the gallon of water to a boil.

➤ Add all the ingredients to the boiling water to bring out the flavor.

➤ Once the mixture has cooled, add it to the remaining water. Note that sandwich bags filled with ice can cool the mixture quickly.

➤ Fully immerse your bird (using a plate to weigh it down, if necessary).

➤ Place in the refrigerator for the appropriate amount of time (4 to 6 hours for a small whole chicken, or up to 12 to 16 hours for a 14-lb. turkey).

➤ After brining, rinse bird well and cook per whatever infusion recipe you have chosen.

➤ Check that the inner thigh temperature is 180° to assure it is fully cooked.

Awesome Asian Bird Brine

Once you have determined how much brine is required to fully immerse your bird, use following the generic brine recipe:

> ➤ 1 gallon water
> ➤ 3 cloves finely chopped garlic
> ➤ ½ finely chopped medium onion
> ➤ 1¼ c. Kosher or Sea salt (or ¾ c. table salt)
> ➤ 1 c. teriyaki or soy sauce
> ➤ ½ c. finely chopped red pepper
> ➤ ¾ c. sugar (or ¾ c. brown sugar)
> ➤ ¼ c. olive oil
> ➤ 1 Tbs. black pepper

Prepping Directions:

> ➤ Follow the prepping directions on page 40.

The Awesome Asian brine recipe yields a Zen hint of eastern culinary subtlety and nicely embellishes such recipes as the Kamikaze Chicken (page 62) the Thai Treat Plucker (page 66), the Maui Wowie Hula Bird (page 114), or the Prancing Peanut Pullet (page 118).

Cluckin' Cajun Cuckoo Bird Brine

Once you have determined how much brine is required to fully immerse your bird, use following the generic brine recipe:

> ➤ 1 gallon water
> ➤ 3 cloves finely chopped garlic cloves
> ➤ ½ finely chopped medium onion
> ➤ 1¼ c. Kosher or Sea salt (or ¾ c. table salt)
> ➤ ¾ c. sugar (or ¾ c brown sugar)
> ➤ ½ c. finely chopped habanero pepper
> ➤ ¼ c. olive oil
> ➤ ¼ c. Tabasco (or hot pepper) sauce
> ➤ 1 Tbs. black pepper
> ➤ ½ Tbs. ground cayenne pepper

Prepping Directions:

➤ Follow the prepping directions on page 40.

The Cluckin' Cajun Cuckoo Bird Brine nicely enhances infusion recipes containing a Cajun-like or spicy theme. Try it with the Très Amigos Chicken (page 58), the Caribbean Jerk Clucker (page 86), the Curried Red Chili Rooster (page 122), the Chipotle Chicken Roast (page 138), or the Cajun Blackened Chicken Roast (page 142).

The Essence of Europe Ballyhoo Bird Brine

Once you have determined how much brine is required to fully immerse your bird, use following the generic brine recipe:

> ➢ 1 gallon water
> ➢ 3 cloves finely chopped garlic
> ➢ ½ finely chopped medium onion
> ➢ 1¼ c. Kosher or Sea salt (or ¾ c. table salt)
> ➢ ¾ c. sugar (or ¾ c brown sugar)
> ➢ ¼ c. olive oil
> ➢ ¼ c. dry white or red wine
> ➢ ¼ c. fresh chopped basil
> ➢ 1 Tbs. oregano
> ➢ 1 Tbs. black pepper
> ➢ ½ Tbs. ground cayenne pepper

Prepping Directions:

➢ Follow the prepping directions on page 40.

The Ballyhoo Bird Brine nicely enhances and brings out the old-world flavor associated with the Cosa Nostra Cuckoo (page 70), the Portuguese Prancing Pullet (page 90), the Chicken à la Dijon (page 94), the Chicken à l'Orange (page 98), or the Chicken Normandy (page 102).

Inject That Bird

In addition to the flavor enhancements of brining comes another technique for introducing flavor into your favorite infusion cooked clucker.

Rubs, sauces, marinades and infusion cooking flavor the bird from the outside in. Injecting flavor deep into the meat can infuse the flavor throughout the bird.

Use a large syringe with a large needle. Purchase a pre-packaged injector kit from your nearest grilling supply shop and save the injector for future uses.

Remember that when injecting, you are delivering flavor to the core of the meat. Be careful not to over-flavor. You want to enhance the natural flavors of your bird...not overpower them.

The following recipes are tried and true injectable sauce concoctions. Try injecting with brining. After the continuous infusion process of cooking, you will be left an amazingly flavorful, juicy and tender bird. Your dinner guests will be stunned and rendered giddy in their utter helplessness by the sheer wonders of such a culinary creation.

Experiment with the various injectable sauce recipes and try mixing and matching with the various poultry recipes presented in this book. Remember that the path to Zen creativity and amazing food is paved by the courageous combination of variables, choices, a fresh bird and your continuous infusion cooker.

Enjoy!

Injection Directions, Tips and Toodles

➤ Take care not to overpower the flavor of the bird with your injectable sauce concoction.

➤ Create your injectable sauce a day before your intent to inject to allow the flavor of your concoction to mingle, socialize and gear up to work their flavor magic.

➤ When injecting the various parts of your bird, inject straight into the center of the meat, withdraw the needle slightly, then re-insert at a 45 ° angle from the original hole on one side, followed by the other. The intent is to inject a bit of flavor throughout the meat center, rather than have pockets of flavor in one place.

➤ Inject the same amount of your injectable sauce concoction during each injection to assure a uniform flavor distribution.

➤ Make sure your injectable sauce concoction is free of "chunks" of herbs and/or vegetable matter to avoid clogging the needle.

➤ Place the needle into the middle of the thick parts of the legs, thighs and breasts.

➤ Coat the rubber part of the plunger in olive oil to assure a good seal.

Injection Quantities

➤ As a rule of thumb, inject approximately 1.5 to 2 ounces of your delectable injectable sauce concoction per lb. of bird.

➤ Measure out your sauce amount into a clean container to inject from. Most of the injectable syringes are graduated so you can use them to measure out your sauce quantities.

➤ Inject into the deepest parts of the thighs, legs and breasts until all of the pre-measured injection sauce concoction is used up.

➤ After injection, clean your syringe and needle well and store for re-use.

Happy Chicken Injection Sauce

The Secret Ingredients

- ½ lb. butter
- 6 oz. beer
- 2 Tbs. Kosher or Sea salt
- 2 Tbs. Worcestershire sauce
- 2 Tbs. soy sauce
- 2 Tbs. garlic powder
- 2 Tbs. finely ground black pepper

Prepping Directions:

- Combine all ingredients in a saucepan over a low heat.
- Stir and heat until all ingredients are mixed evenly.
- Enhance the flavor by refrigerating for 24 hours prior to injecting.
- Over low heat, re-warm injectable sauce concoction.
- Inject as instructed on page 45 prior to cooking.

Cajun Creole Injectable Delight
The Secret Ingredients

- ½ lb. butter
- ¼ c. cider vinegar
- 1 Tbs. cayenne pepper
- 1 Tbs. black pepper
- 1 Tbs. garlic powder
- 1 Tbs. paprika
- 3 Tbs. cayenne pepper sauce
- 1 Tbs. Worcestershire sauce
- 1 ½ Tbs. Kosher or Sea salt
- 1 tsp. ground cumin
- ½ tsp. basil
- ½ tsp. oregano
- 12 oz. of a robust dark beer

Prepping Directions:

- Combine all ingredients in a saucepan over a low heat.
- Stir and heat until all ingredients are mixed evenly.
- Enhance the flavor by refrigerating for 24 hours prior to injecting.
- Over low heat, re-warm injectable sauce concoction.
- Inject as instructed on page 45 prior to cooking.

Caribbean Tango Injectable Marinade

The Secret Ingredients

- ½ c. lime juice
- ¼ c. olive oil
- ¼ c. powdered sugar
- 1 Tbs. ginger powder
- 1 Tbs. ground cayenne pepper
- 1 Tbs. ground black pepper
- 1 Tbs. garlic powder
- 1 tsp. cinnamon
- 1 tsp. onion powder

Prepping Directions:

- Combine all ingredients in a saucepan over a low heat.
- Stir and heat until all ingredients are mixed evenly.
- Enhance the flavor by refrigerating for 24 hours prior to injecting.
- Over low heat, re-warm injectable sauce concoction.
- Inject as instructed on page 45 prior to cooking.

Czar Nick's Injection Sauce

- 2 c. vodka
- 1 c. cranberry juice
- 1 c. apple juice
- ½ c. olive oil
- ¼ lb. butter
- 1 Tbs. honey
- 1 Tbs. garlic powder
- 1 Tbs. paprika
- 2 tsp. onion powder

Prepping Directions:

- Combine all ingredients in a saucepan over a low heat.
- Stir and heat until all ingredients are mixed evenly.
- Enhance the flavor by refrigerating for 24 hours prior to injecting.
- Over low heat, re-warm injectable sauce concoction.
- Inject as instructed on page 45 prior to cooking.

Firewater Fizzle Injection Sauce

- ➢ 2 c. Kentucky bourbon
- ➢ 1 c. vodka
- ➢ 1 c. cream soda
- ➢ ½ c. olive oil
- ➢ ½ c. Worcestershire sauce
- ➢ ¼ lb. butter
- ➢ 1 Tbs. garlic powder
- ➢ 1 Tbs. ground black pepper
- ➢ 1½ tsp. Kosher or Sea salt

Prepping Directions:

- ➢ Combine all ingredients in a saucepan over a low heat.
- ➢ Stir and heat until all ingredients are mixed evenly.
- ➢ Enhance the flavor by refrigerating for 24 hours prior to injecting.
- ➢ Over low heat, re-warm injectable sauce concoction.
- ➢ Inject as instructed on page 45 prior to cooking.

The Zen of Beer and Other Liquid Libations

There is an unlimited choice of flavor liquids that can be used in the flavor bases of the infusion cookers. Imagination and creativity are the main requirements!

12 to 15 oz. of your flavor concoction added to each infusion cooker's flavor base is all that is needed. For the Poultry Pal®, fill the base itself. For the Vertical Chicken Roaster and the Chickāno, fill the flavor towers until they overflow into the base. With the Chickāno, use a supporting casserole or pie dish as a base to catch the excess liquid libations.

Wines, fruit juices and various soda pops can also impart distinctive and subtle flavor to the bird. We have tried everything from root beer to chicken broth, which can be used as delicious gravy or soup base after the bird has been cooked. Your imagination and creativity are the only limitations!

Once you have chosen your flavor liquid, feel free to embellish it with more spices. A handful of garlic, a couple of teaspoons of lemon pepper and/or some chili powder sprinkled into the liquid can add unique and infinite subtleties of flavor to the bird. Be creative!

You can even throw in a handful of vegetables to the flavor broth such as small red potatoes, celery, onion or others for later addition to sautés or soup stocks.

Or try any of the brines and injectable concoction suggestions for even greater creative flexibility.

Zen Chicken Recipes and the Art of Continuous Infusion

The following recipes are tried and true. They reflect the incredible creative potential and infinite variety possible by cooking chicken using the continuous infusion method. Try these recipes and let us know how they work for you...or come up with your own. Note that all the recipes list temperature in degrees F.

You can give us feedback or share an original recipe at:

www.redowlpublications.com

Enjoy, be creative, dance a jig and smile a lot. Enjoy your creation with friends and family. Remember the Zen path of balance, creativity and harmony, easily found and enjoyed through the continuous infusion cooking process.

Bon Appétit!

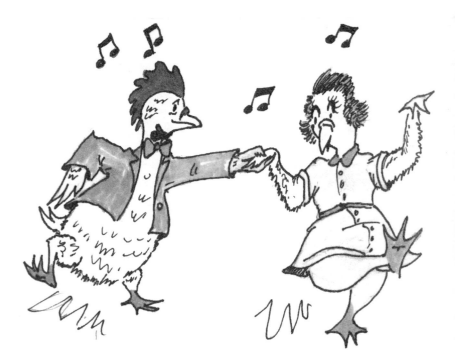

Zen and the Art of...

Kansas City Bar-B-Que Bird

Ah yes…the traditional Barbecue chicken. The poultry politic, grilled and eaten across this great country of ours. Eliciting passion, controversy and full, satisfied bellies amongst the Barbecue traditionalists from Kansas to Texas.

Kansas City Bar-B-Que Bird

Basic Stuff

1 3 to 6 lb. chicken
½ c. vegetable or olive oil
1 c. barbecue sauce

Rub

2 Tbs. brown sugar
2 Tbs. sweet or hot paprika
1 Tbs. Kosher or Sea salt
1 Tbs. chili powder
1 Tbs. garlic powder
1 Tbs. ground pepper to taste

Liquid Flavor Essence

32 oz. of fine dark beer

Cooking Directions:

➤ Place bird on flavor tower.

➤ Using a basting brush liberally paint the chicken with the liquid flavor base.

➤ Generously apply the rub to the outside and the cavity of the bird.

➤ Add the beer to the flavor base.

➤ In a conventional oven, cook at 350° for 1½ to 2 hours or until the drippings are clear and the leg quarters move easily in their joints.

➤ Using a basting brush, paint the bird with your Barbecue Sauce about an hour into the cooking.

➤ Drink the remaining 24 oz. of beer while the bird is cooking.

➤ If grilling, follow the indirect heating method as explained on page 25.

➤ Remove cooked chicken from grill or oven, let stand five minutes and serve.

Serve with some coleslaw, baked beans, biscuits and fresh corn on the cob. Be sure to have plenty of beer handy and avoid any discussions regarding politics, religions or favorite football teams. Enjoy the sunlight, the fresh breeze and the laughter of friends as you share this fine traditional American meal.

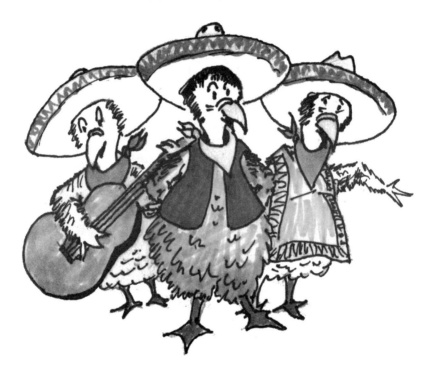

Zen and the Art of...

Trés Amigos Chicken

The Trés Amigos chicken brings out some special flavor á la Mexicana. Trés Amigos means Three Friends...Our three friends in this case are Mole, Tequila and Señor Chicken. Mole sauce is an old Mexican favorite and provides a unique flavor with a hint of chocolate merged with spice. The mole sauce needs to be prepared first. I have provided a quick microwave-based recipe for the sauce. Note that this recipe calls for a lower temperature and longer cook time. An aluminum tent is recommended. The mole sauce is prone to burning, so care must be taken. Have fun with this one and Olé!

Trés Amigos Chicken

Basic Stuff

1 3 to 6 lb. chicken
1 c. Mole sauce (see page 35)
½ c. vegetable or extra virgin olive oil

Liquid Flavor Essence

6 oz. of tequila
6 oz. of a light colored Mexican beer
A pinch of garlic powder
A pinch of cumin
A pinch of chili powder

Cooking Directions

➤ Place bird on flavor tower.
➤ Using a basting brush liberally paint the chicken with the liquid flavor base.
➤ Add the ingredients for the liquid flavor essence to the flavor base.
➤ In a conventional oven, cook at 325° for 1 ½ to 2 hours or until the drippings are clear and the leg quarters move easily in their joints.
➤ After 45 minutes, begin basting the bird with the mole sauce every 15 minutes or so until done.
➤ If grilling, follow the indirect heating method as explained on page 25.
➤ Using an aluminum tent with this recipe is a good idea to prevent the mole glaze from burning. If desired, use the aluminum tent once you start basting with the mole. Discard in the last 15 minutes of cooking.
➤ Remove chicken from grill and sprinkle with cilantro.

This bird is great served with a fresh salad sprinkled with cilantro and tortilla chips, corn on the cob and a margarita or two to wash it all down in style and with great social camaraderie! For dessert, add vanilla ice cream covered with grated chocolate and served with cinnamon-toasted tortillas.

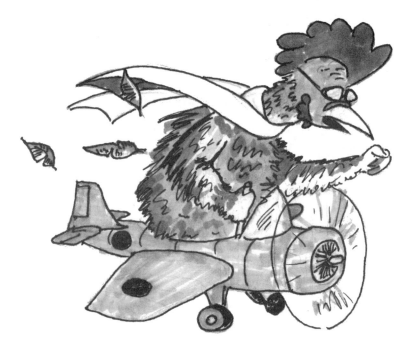

Zen and the Art of...

Kamikaze Chicken

We have always enjoyed the subtle and simple flavor associated with Japanese cuisine. Therein lies a certain Zen quality to living simply and elegantly yet with unbridled gusto and zest, akin to enjoying a rock garden or praising the simple form of a Bonsai tree. Here is a recipe for a wonderful Japanese approach to a happy Samurai bird and Zen harmony at your dinner table. Enjoy!

Kamikaze Chicken

Basic Stuff

1 3 to 5 lb. chicken
½ c. sesame seed oil

Rub

2 tsp. Wasabe powder
2 tsp. sesame seeds
1 tsp. Kosher or Sea Salt
1 tsp. black pepper
1 tsp. powdered ginger
1 tsp. garlic powder

Liquid Flavor Essence

6 oz. sake
4 oz. rice vinegar
2 oz. teriyaki sauce
A pinch of garlic powder
A pinch of Wasabe powder (available
in the gourmet section of your supermarket)

Cooking Directions:

➤ Place bird on flavor tower.

➤ Using a basting brush liberally paint the chicken with the liquid flavor base.

➤ Generously apply the rub to the outside and the cavity of the bird.

➤ Add the ingredients for the liquid flavor essence to the flavor base.

➤ In a conventional oven, cook at 350° for 1¼ to 1½ hours or until the drippings are clear and the leg quarters move easily in their joints.

➤ If grilling, follow the indirect heating method as explained on page 25.

➤ Remove chicken from grill or oven, let stand 5 minutes, garnish with thinly sliced strips of Daikon radish, cucumber slices and fresh baby carrots.

Serve with a fresh salad, firm asparagus seasoned with teriyaki sauce and sesame seeds, fresh steamed whole soybeans in the pod and warm sake. A glass of plum wine will make for a nice dessert.

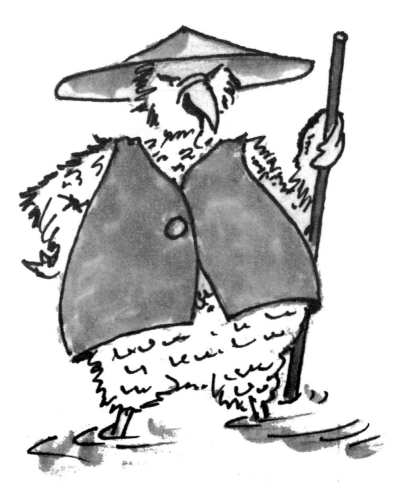

Zen and the Art of...

Thai Treat Plucker

Thai cooking is unique in its combination of sweet and hot. The essence of the South Pacific can make for a refreshing change and delight the palate as well. The key to the Thai Treat Chicken is the sweetness of coconut milk mingled with the spice of red pepper. If you are not into spice, forego the red pepper or spice accordingly to taste.

Thai Treat Plucker

Basic Stuff
1 3 to 6 lb. chicken
1 13.5 oz. can coconut milk
½ c. grated coconut
Peanut oil

Rub
2 tsp. ginger powder
1 tsp. lemon zest
1 tsp. Kosher or Sea Salt
2 tsp. garlic powder
1 tsp. ground hot red pepper

Liquid Flavor Essence:
10 oz. coconut milk
4 oz. lemon juice
A pinch of garlic powder
A pinch of ground ginger
A pinch of lemon zest

Cooking Directions:

➤ Place bird on flavor tower.

➤ Take ½ cup of the liquid flavor essence and set aside as basting sauce.

➤ Using a basting brush liberally paint bird with peanut oil and generously apply rub.

➤ Add the ingredients for liquid flavor essence to flavor base.

➤ In a conventional oven, cook at 325° for 1½ to 2 hours or until the drippings are clear and the leg quarters move easily in their joints. After 45 minutes of cooking, baste bird with the basting sauce every ten to 15 minutes until cooked.

➤ If grilling, follow the indirect heating method as explained on page 25.

➤ Remove from oven or grill and let stand 5 minutes.

➤ Baste once more with the basting sauce and liberally sprinkle finely shredded coconut over bird.

Serve with a fresh salad, a medley of snow peas, onions and bamboo shoots quickly sautéed in white wine. Present each dinner guest a cup of steamed white rice as a final touch to an awesome meal.

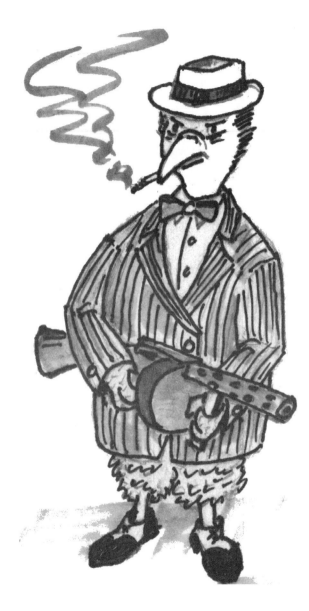

Zen and the Art of...

Cosa Nostra Cuckoo

From the open countryside and quaint villages of Sicily comes another excursion into the wonders of cuckoo culinary delights. Here is a chicken recipe that can't be refused! Be careful with this recipe as it has long been considered a family secret and you don't want to end up sleeping with the chickens! Try it and enjoy. If life's trials begin to stress you and Vito wants his cash, fuhgedduhboutit! After all…"Whaddaya gonna do"? Make some great chow and drink to your paisson's longevity...Capiche?

Cosa Nostra Cuckoo

Basic Stuff

1 3 to 6 lb. chicken
½ c. extra virgin olive oil

Rub

2 tsp. ground rosemary
2 tsp. garlic powder
1 tsp. oregano

Liquid Flavor Essence

12 oz. of a dry Merlot or Chianti wine

Cooking Directions:

➤ Place bird on flavor tower.

➤ Using a basting brush, paint the critter with the olive oil and generously apply the rub.

➤ Add the wine and any remaining rub into the flavor base.

➤ In a conventional oven, cook at 350° for 1¼ to 1½ hours or until the drippings are clear and the leg quarters move easily in their joints.

➤ If grilling, follow the indirect heating method as explained on page 25.

➤ Remove cooked chicken from grill or oven, let stand five minutes and garnish with baby carrots and broccoli cuttings.

Serve with some antipasto, a fresh salad, some fine dry red wine, red potatoes with capers and ricotta stuffed Portabella mushrooms. A fine cognac will make for a great finale after this wonderful meal.

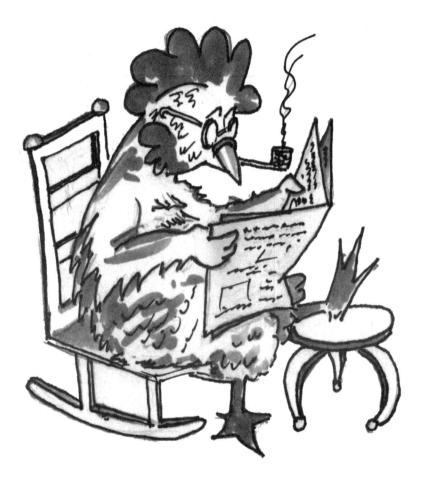

Zen and the Art of...

Grandpa Tom's Homestyle Bird

A full chicken meal perfect for warming the soul and the belly when you've worked hard and it's cold outside. Rib sticking, fire in the fireplace, a cold wind blowin' outside is the theme for this down home recipe. Close your eyes; you can almost hear the snow fall and the dog snore.

Grandpa Tom's Homestyle Bird

Basic Stuff

1 3 to 6 lb. chicken
½ c. vegetable or olive oil

Rub:

2 Tbs. Kosher or Sea Salt
2 Tbs. ground oregano
2 Tbs. garlic powder
1 Tbs. dried rosemary
Ground pepper to taste

Liquid Flavor Essence:

12 oz. chicken broth

Cooking Directions:

➤ Place bird on flavor tower.

➤ Using a basting brush, paint the critter with the olive oil and generously apply the rub.

➤ Add the chicken broth to the flavor base. You may use canned or make your own from bouillon. Spice broth to taste.

➤ If desired, line the base of the chicken with red potatoes, whole carrots and onion slices.

➤ In a conventional oven, cook at 350° for 1¼ to 1½ hours or until the drippings are clear and the leg quarters move easily in their joints.

➤ If grilling, follow the indirect heating method as explained on page 25.

➤ The liquid from the flavor base can now be used as an awesome base for gravy poured over the chicken cooked veggies and/or as soup base for extending the leftovers into another new meal.

Serve chicken with the red spud, carrot and onion medley covered in gravy (made from the flavor base stock of course!), a fresh salad, biscuits or rolls and generous helpings of broccoli in cheese sauce. A warmed apple pie with a dollop of vanilla ice cream over the top will fully complete this down-home culinary dance. Enjoy, stay warm, smile a lot and be good to your neighbors!

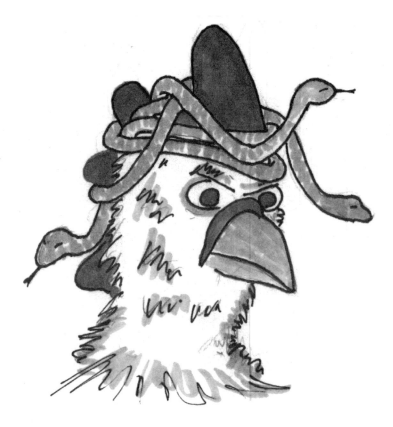

Zen and the Art of...

Uncle Jerry's Medusa Apple Chicken

An enticing chicken meal, perfect for warming the soul and tickling the fancy of even the most hard-to-please rapscallions. Greek mythology always claimed that all mortals would be turned to stone if their eyes gazed directly upon the Medusa. Uncle Jerry has come up with a Medusa creation using apples and imagination. Fear not, this delectable will not turn you to stone or any other type of hard, inorganic substance! It will tickle your taste buds and titillate your flavor nodules...setting them to quivering with a unique and visually silly approach to cooking chicken. With apple slices sticking out of the neck hole, this lil' beastie may look like a Medusa but it tastes like a dream of peace in a field of fruit and whipped cream. Enjoy!

Uncle Jerry's Medusa Apple Chicken

Basic Stuff
1 3 to 6 lb. chicken
1 cored and sliced apple
½ c. vegetable oil

Rub:
3 Tbs. cinnamon
2 Tbs. brown sugar
1 Tbs. Kosher or Sea Salt
1 Tbs. ground cloves

Liquid Flavor Essence:
12 oz. apple juice

Cooking Directions:

➤ Stuff an apple core into the top of the flavor tower. Place bird onto the flavor tower. Stuff apple wedges into the neck-hole at the top of the chicken in a radial fashion.

➤ Using a basting brush, paint the critter with vegetable oil and generously apply the rub.

➤ Add the apple juice to the flavor base. Throw the leftover rub into the flavor base for good measure.

➤ In a conventional oven, cook at 350° for 1¼ to 1½ hours or until the drippings are clear and the leg quarters move easily in their joints.

➤ If grilling, follow the indirect heating method as explained on page 25.

➤ Remove cooked chicken from grill or oven and let stand.

➤ If desired, pour a little warmed maple syrup over the bird and apple slices.

Serve chicken with a fresh salad, a generous serving of the vegetables of your choice, some bread and a fine white wine and end with chocolate mousse laced with brandy. There will be no stones left here!

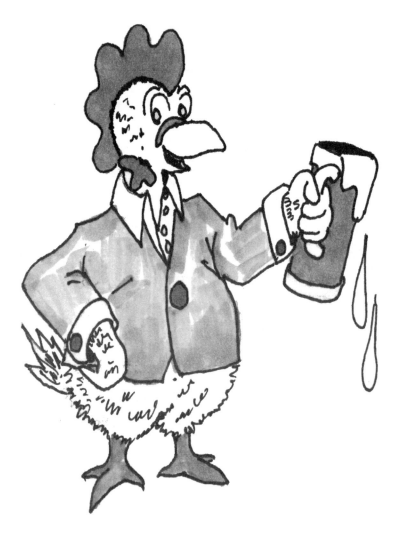

Zen and the Art of...

Belfast Blarney Spud Bird

"There once was a chicken from Derry,
Who hopped around blissful and merry.
With the Poultry Pal's tower,
He'd be cooked in an hour
With a taste and a texture quite scary."

Indeed, this Irish delight will combine the lightness of potato with a hint of oak-aged whiskey to create a bird which will engender the spontaneous generation of limericks and a plethora of blarney around the table and out into the streets. Watch out for the leprechauns with this one!

Belfast Blarney Spud Bird

Basic Stuff
1 3 to 5 lb. chicken
½ c. ranch salad dressing
1 c. instant potato flakes

Rub
1 tsp. Kosher or Sea Salt
1 tsp. black pepper
1 tsp. garlic powder

Liquid Flavor Essence
6 oz. Irish whiskey
6 oz. dark beer

Cooking Directions:

➤ Using a basting brush liberally paint the chicken with the ranch dressing.

➤ Sprinkle the rub over the ranch dressing.

➤ Roll the bird in a pan containing the instant potato flakes.

➤ Add the ingredients for the liquid flavor essence to the flavor base.

➤ Line the base of the flavor tower with small red potatoes and chunks of cubed onion.

➤ In a conventional oven, cook at 350° for 1¼ to 1½ hours or until the drippings are clear and the leg quarters move easily in their joints.

➤ If grilling, follow the indirect heating method as explained on page 25.

➤ Remove Blarney Bird from the grill or oven and let stand 5 minutes.

Serve with a fine dark beer, fresh salad and green beans spiced with dill weed. The luck of the Irish and charms of the leprechauns will permeate your dinner table. Be careful however; you may find your diners suddenly spouting limericks and quickly leaving the table to find green socks and 4-leaf clovers.

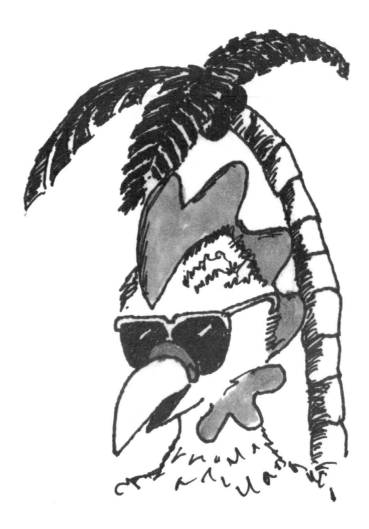

Zen and the Art of...

Caribbean Jerk Clucker

The essence of Caribbean cuisine lies in the combination of sweet and hot. This sweet spicy clucker will conjure images of warm oceans on hot beaches echoing with the sounds of calypso melody and rhythms. You will find yourself dreaming of lazy days, warm souls and the sweetness of Piña Coladas imbibed on the beach. Resist the urge to tango until after eating this Caribbean Clucking Creation, for it has been shown that doing the tango while eating can be disruptive to good digestion. Flavor the bird with the spices of the Caribbean and then complete the cooking by locking in those tango-laden flavors with a sweet-hot Jamaican glaze. Delight in the essence of sun, surf and hot wild nights!

Caribbean Jerk Clucker

Basic Stuff

1 3 to 5 lb. chicken
2¼ c. Caribbean Jerk Glaze (page 36)
½ c. olive oil

Rub

2 tsp. garlic powder
1 tsp. Kosher or Sea Salt
1 tsp. onion powder
1 tsp. cayenne powder
½ tsp. allspice
½ tsp. cinnamon
¼ tsp. nutmeg

Liquid Flavor Essence

6 oz. dark rum
6 oz. lime juice

Cooking Directions

➤ Make the Caribbean Jerk Glaze (see page 36).
➤ Using a basting brush liberally paint the chicken with the glaze.
➤ Roll the bird in a pan containing the rub and generously coat the bird.
➤ Add the ingredients for the liquid flavor essence to the flavor base.
➤ Line the base of the flavor tower with mandarin oranges, chunks of mango and cubed onion.
➤ In a conventional oven, cook at 350° for 1¼ to 1½ hours or until the drippings are clear and the leg quarters move easily in their joints.
➤ If grilling, follow the indirect heating method as explained on page 25.
➤ Remove from grill and let stand 5 minutes prior to carving.

Serve with shrimp sautéed with mangos, mandarin orange slices, onion, garlic and hot peppers in a rum laden mixture of soy and leftover glaze. Spice to taste, using the Habanero pepper sauce. Habanero peppers are very hot but have a wonderful flavor perfect to mix with the Caribbean sweetness. Enjoy with a fine rum beverage, a fire on the beach and smiles of good friends.

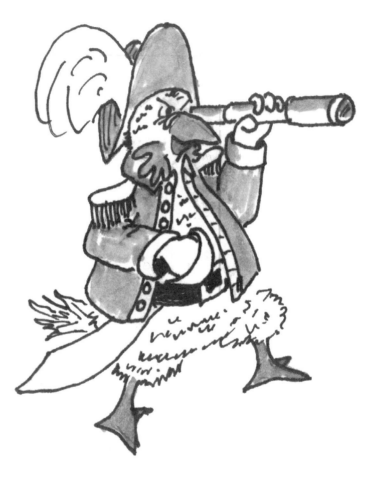

Zen and the Art of...

Portuguese Prancing Pullet

This recipe visits the elegance of Portuguese cuisine. This cuckoo concoction spontaneously elicits images of old sailing ships and courageous explorations of a square world from which one could fall off if sailing too close to the edge. Cook this pullet and lose yourself in visions of the Old World, the sounds of seagulls, the washing of the surf and the warmth of friends and family. Know that getting close to the edge can be a thrilling experience. Enjoy! And man the masts with enthusiasm!

Portuguese Prancing Pullet

Basic Stuff
1 3 to 5 lb. chicken
1 c. chopped green peppers
1 c. chopped red peppers
½ c. capers
½ c. olive oil
1 dozen small Portabella mushrooms

Rub
1 tsp. Kosher or Sea Salt
1 tsp. black pepper
1 tsp. garlic powder

Liquid Flavor Essence
12 oz. of Madeira wine

Cooking Directions

➤ Using a basting brush, liberally paint the chicken with the olive oil and apply the rub.

➤ Add the Madeira wine to the flavor base.

➤ Line the base of the flavor tower with peppers, capers and mushrooms.

➤ In a conventional oven, cook at 350° for 1¼ to 1½ hours or until the drippings are clear and the leg quarters move easily in their joints.

➤ If grilling, follow the indirect heating method as explained on page 25.

➤ Remove the sea-faring pullet from the grill or oven and let stand 5 minutes.

➤ If desired, make gravy out of the remaining liquid in the flavor base with flour and milk to add zest to the chicken and vegetables.

Serve with a fine dry red wine, a fresh salad, rice seasoned with the Madeira gravy, an olive oil-sautéed mixture of garlic cloves, baby carrots, onion and green peppers and warm bread with tarragon-seasoned butter. The elegance and Old World charm of this lavish bird will keep your diners rapt in culinary maritime bliss.

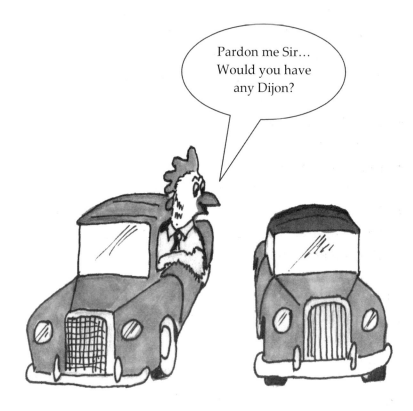

Chicken à la Dijon

This recipe, borrowed from the elegance of fine French cuisine, incorporates the gentle spiciness of Dijon mustard with the clean dryness of a fine Chardonnay. This cuckoo creation conjures images of small cafés exuding Old World charm along the sidewalks of Paris. This bird's delicate flavor will conjure images of Parisian streets echoing with festive music, artisan displays and the aroma of the street Bistros. There is nothing like the essence of Old World Paris ambiance, fine wine, warm days and lively evenings. Bon Appétit!

Chicken à la Dijon

Basic Stuff
1 3 to 5 lb. chicken
1 c. chopped green peppers
1 c. chopped red peppers
½ c. capers
½ c. olive oil
1 dozen small Portabella mushrooms

Rub
¼ c. Dijon mustard
1 Tbs. brown sugar
1 tsp. Kosher or Sea Salt
1 tsp. tarragon
1 tsp. garlic powder

Liquid Flavor Essence
12 oz. of dry Chardonnay

Cooking Directions

➤ Make the rub by mixing the rub ingredients, throwing in a splash of olive oil and a splash of Chardonnay to desired consistency.

➤ Using a basting brush, liberally paint the chicken with the olive oil and apply the rub.

➤ Add the Chardonnay wine to the flavor base.

➤ Line the base of the flavor tower with slices onions and mushrooms.

➤ In a conventional oven, cook at 325 to 350° for 1¼ to 1½ hours or until the drippings are clear and the leg quarters move easily in their joints.

➤ If grilling, follow the indirect heating method as explained on page 25.

➤ Remove Monsieur Chicken from the grill or oven and let stand 5 minutes.

Serve with a fine wine of your choice, a fresh salad, French bread and a sautéed mixture of broccoli, baby carrots, onion and green peppers. The gentle spice of the Dijon will impart a subtle and distinctive flavor to this French delight.

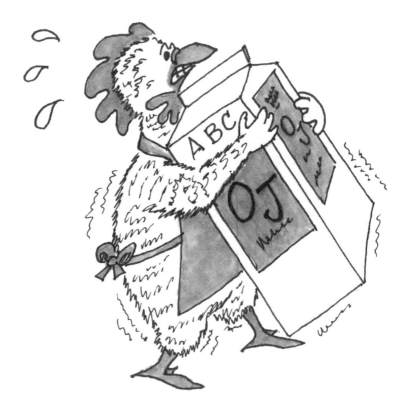

Zen and the Art of...

Chicken à l'Orange

Chicken à l'Orange incorporates the subtle yet distinct essence of citrus and a hint of warm days in basking sun. Mom used to say you have to eat your fruit. All that Vitamin C and good stuff will keep you strong to resist colds. If Linus Pauling were alive today, he would most assuredly endorse this fruity clucker. So call the kids, whip out the oranges and rock into a healthy, fruity and sweet cuckoo contrivance.

Chicken à l'Orange

Basic Stuff
1 3 to 5 lb. chicken
1 dozen small Portabella mushrooms
1 c. chopped green peppers
1 c. chopped red peppers
½ c. lime juice
½ c. olive oil
½ c. capers

Rub
1 tsp. Kosher or Sea Salt
1 tsp. black pepper
1 tsp. garlic powder

Liquid Flavor Essence
12 oz. of orange juice

Cooking Directions

➤ Make the rub by mixing the rub ingredients, throwing in a splash of olive oil and a splash of orange juice to the desired consistency.

➤ Using a basting brush, liberally paint the chicken with the olive oil and apply the rub.

➤ Add the liquid essence to the flavor base.

➤ Line the base of the flavor tower with slices of onions and mushrooms.

➤ In a conventional oven, cook at 350° for 1¼ to 1½ hours or until the drippings are clear and the leg quarters move easily in their joints.

➤ If grilling, follow the indirect heating method as explained on page 25.

➤ Remove Monsieur Chicken from the grill or oven and let stand 5 minutes.

Serve with a fine wine of your choice, a fresh salad and a sautéed mixture of broccoli, baby carrots, onion and green peppers. May the essence of gay Paris permeate your kitchen and your dinner table! Nous sommes du soleil!

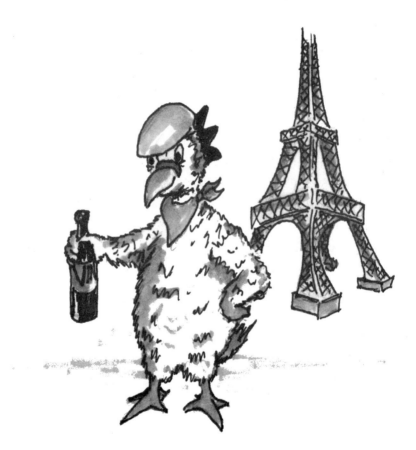

Zen and the Art of...

Chicken Normandy

From the north of France comes a cuckoo concoction using the essence of apples and brandy to titillate even the most discerning palates. This dish presents a hint of fruity sweetness combined with the elegance of a delicately cooked chicken. Your dinner guests will be amazed and some may even start speaking in French aphorisms as the concoction is enthusiastically consumed.

Chicken Normandy

Basic Stuff
1 3 to 6 lb. chicken
1 onion chopped
1 c. peeled and sliced apple
1 c. sliced mushrooms
½ c. vegetable or extra virgin olive oil
¼ c. butter

Rub
2 Tbs. Kosher or Sea Salt
2 Tbs. pepper
1 Tbs. garlic powder
1 Tbs. ground thyme

Liquid Flavor Essence
1 c. brandy
¾ c. apple juice

Cooking Directions

➢ Place bird on flavor tower.

➢ Using a basting brush, paint the critter with the olive oil and generously apply the rub.

➢ Add all of the liquid flavor essence to the flavor base of the cooker.

➢ In a conventional oven, cook at 350° for 1½ hours or until the drippings are clear and the leg quarters move easily in their joints.

➢ If grilling, follow the indirect heating method as explained on page 25.

➢ Sauté the mushrooms, apple and onions in the butter until tender.

➢ Remove cooked chicken from the cooker and set aside.

➢ Make the Gravy à La Normandy out of the drippings (page 36).

➢ Coat the sautéed mixture with a dollop of the gravy. Mix up and serve.

Serve with a lightly tossed fresh salad, some boiled red potatoes and a good loaf of fresh French bread to soak up the gravy. Drink to the health of your family and guests knowing that they have just eaten an amazing culinary cuckoo concoction fit for the court of Louis XIV and your family and friends.

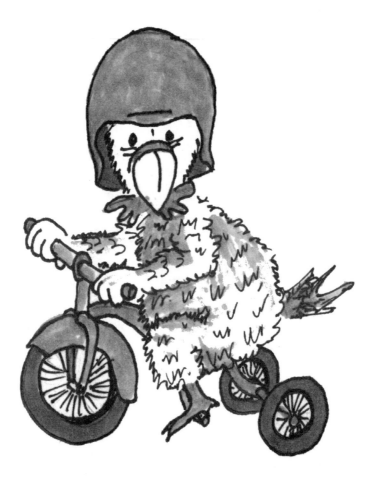

Zen and the Art of...

Bavarian Kraut Bird

This chicken delectable is borrowed from the hills and country of central Germany. This recipe is served up with the Prussian taste for kielbasa and sauerkraut. This creation conjures up images of mid-winter warmth when the fire in the fireplace is warming hearts and home, the temperature is crunchy-cold outside and the forest is quiet, resplendent in its Germanic winter cover.

Bavarian Kraut Bird

Basic Stuff

1 3 to 6 lb. chicken
1 2-foot long kielbasa sausage
1 onion chopped
1 c. prepared sauerkraut
½ c. vegetable or extra virgin olive oil

Rub

2 Tbs. Kosher or Sea Salt
2 Tbs. pepper
1 Tbs. garlic powder

Liquid Flavor Essence

12 to 15 oz. of a fine Hefenweizen (wheat) beer

Cooking Directions

➤ Place bird on flavor tower.

➤ Using a basting brush, paint the critter with the olive oil and generously apply the rub.

➤ Add 12 to 15 oz. of the Hefenweizen liquid flavor essence to the flavor base of the cooker.

➤ Place the flavor tower on the base and roll the Kielbasa sausage around the outside edge of the flavor base.

➤ Using the sauerkraut and onion, make a nest at the base of the chicken between the bird and the sausage.

➤ In a conventional oven, cook at 350° for 1½ hours or until the drippings are clear and the leg quarters move easily in their joints.

➤ If grilling, follow the indirect heating method as explained on page 25.

Serve with mashed potatoes, some green beans and fresh dinner rolls. An apéritif of genuine Schnapps with bold toasts to family and friends will make this Bavarian Kraut bird a meal to remember.

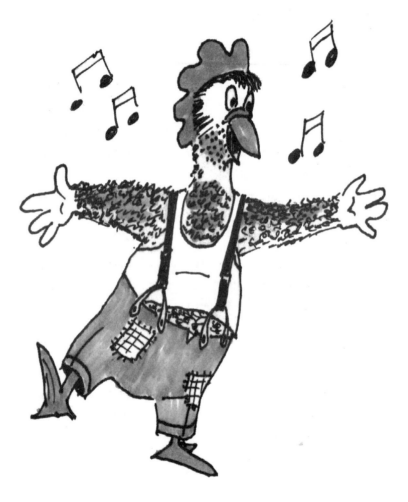

Zen and the Art of...

Zorba's Zesty Squawker

From the island of Greece came the platitudes of Plato, the sensibility of Socrates, the arrogance of Apollo and the Zestiness of Zorba's Squawking Zen-bird. This delicacy was the food of the athletes as they performed in the Olympiad…and it is said that even Zeus had a weakness for this delectable, granting immortality to any mortal who would prepare such a dish as an offering to the Gods.

Zorba's Zesty Squawker

Basic Stuff

1 3 to 6 lb. chicken
1 c. whole green olives
1 c. mushrooms
1 c. crumbled feta cheese
½ c. vegetable or extra virgin olive oil

Rub

2 Tbs. Kosher or Sea Salt
2 Tbs. pepper
1 Tbs. garlic powder
¼ c. fresh basil
¼ c. fresh oregano
¼ c. fresh thyme

Liquid Flavor Essence

12 to 15 oz. of Marsala wine

Cooking Directions

➤ Place bird on flavor tower.

➤ Using a basting brush, paint the critter with the olive oil and generously apply the rub.

➤ Add 12 to 15 oz. of the Marsala wine liquid flavor essence to the flavor base of the cooker.

➤ Place the olives and mushrooms liberally around the base of the bird and splash with a bit of the Marsala.

➤ In a conventional oven, cook at 350° for 1½ hours or until the drippings are clear and the leg quarters move easily in their joints.

➤ If grilling, follow the indirect heating method as explained on page 25.

➤ Remove cooked bird from the grill or oven and liberally sprinkle with the crumbled feta cheese prior to serving.

Serve with a fresh tossed salad, green beans spiced with dill and hard sourdough bread. Once prepared, sit back and watch the rapture on your guests' faces as they lose themselves in the essence of Greece and the history of humanity.

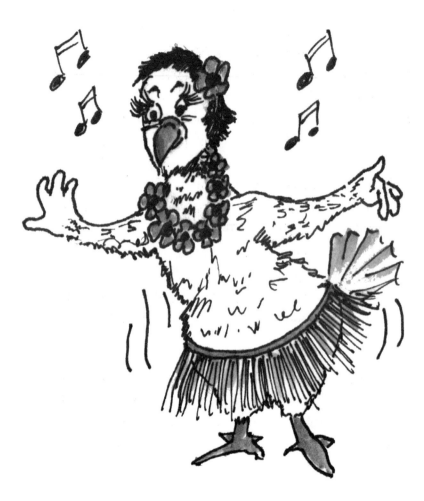

Zen and the Art of...

Maui Wowie Hula Bird

From the islands of Hawaii comes a recipe celebrating the joy and cheer of a fine sunny luau, resplendent with sunshine, warm waves, hula dances and ukuleles strumming up the early evening toasts to friends and family.

Maui Wowie Hula Bird

Basic Stuff
1 3 to 6 lb. chicken
1 c. sliced mango
1 c. shredded coconut
½ c. vegetable or extra virgin olive oil

Rub
2 Tbs. powdered ginger
2 Tbs. garlic powder
2 Tbs. pepper
1 Tbs. Kosher or Sea Salt

Liquid Flavor Essence
8 oz. pineapple juice
4 oz. soy sauce
4 oz. dark rum

Cooking Directions

➤ Place bird on flavor tower.
➤ Line the base of the bird with the sliced mangos and shredded coconut.
➤ Using a basting brush, paint the critter with the olive oil, the liquid flavor essence and then generously apply the rub. Sprinkle with the coconut.
➤ Add the remaining liquid flavor essence to the flavor base of the cooker.
➤ In a conventional oven, cook at 350° for 1½ hours or until the drippings are clear and the leg quarters move easily in their joints.
➤ If grilling, follow the indirect heating method as explained on page 25.

Serve with a fresh fruit salad, fresh peas and dinner rolls. This light meal will lure your senses to innocent contemplation of warm sands, gentle breezes, the sounds of the surf mingling with song and the inescapable of harmony of Hawaiian hospitality.

Aloha!

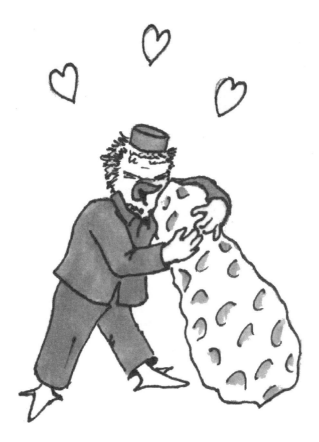

Zen and the Art of...

Prancing Peking Peanut Pullet

From the Great Wall of China to the steppes of Mongolia, the Chinese people have embellished their culinary wisdom with the versatility of the peanut. This simple legume has been a staple to Chinese cooking since it was transported to China via the Philippines by Spanish galleons before 1600. The Chinese folks called peanuts "foreign beans". They spread from there throughout China and to Japan where they are known as "Chinese beans". Chinese settlers were probably responsible for introduction of this poultry-enhancing legume to the rest of Southeast Asia and Indonesia.

Peking Peanut Pullet

Basic Stuff

1 3 to 6 lb. chicken
1 chopped onion
2 c. peanuts
1½ c. Peking Peanut Sauce (page 37)

Liquid Flavor Essence

12 oz. dark beer
4 oz. Soy Sauce

Cooking Directions

- Place bird on flavor tower.
- Line the base of the bird with the peanuts and chopped onion.
- Using a basting brush, paint the critter with the peanut sauce.
- Add the liquid flavor essence to the flavor base of the cooker.
- In a conventional oven, cook at 325° for 1½ hours or until the drippings are clear and the leg quarters move easily in their joints.
- If grilling, follow the indirect heating method as explained on page 25.

Serve with fresh salad, a mixture of snow peapods, bean sprouts and water chestnuts. This meal will awaken the peaceful Zen spirit of the Shaolin monk that lives deep within you and your guests' consciousness. Be at peace and enjoy the moment and the meal in harmony and good energy.

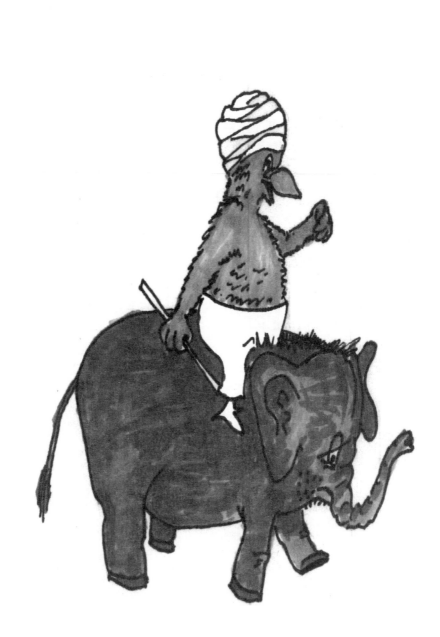

Zen and the Art of...

Curried Red Chili Rooster

This East Asian concoction reflects the cuisine of India. The curry spice mix has always been a staple of Indian cuisine. Reflections of exotic elephants, Bengal tigers and the blessings of Shiva fill this recipe with an elegance and simplicity that will titillate your taste buds.

Curried Red Chili Rooster

Basic Stuff

1 3 to 6 lb. chicken
1 c. extra virgin olive oil

Rub

1 Tbs. Kosher or Sea Salt
2 Tbs. garlic powder
2 Tbs. curry powder
½ tsp. ground cinnamon
½ tsp. ground red pepper
½ tsp. allspice
½ tsp. ground cumin

Liquid Flavor Essence

12 oz. dark beer

Cooking Directions

➤ Using a basting brush, paint the critter with the olive oil.

➤ Roll the bird in a mixture of the rub spices.

➤ Place the bird on the flavor tower.

➤ Add the liquid flavor essence to the flavor base of the cooker.

➤ In a conventional oven, cook at 350° for 1½ hours or until the drippings are clear and the leg quarters move easily in their joints.

➤ If grilling, follow the indirect heating method as explained on page 25.

Serve with black-eyed pea salad, curried rice and dinner rolls. Enjoy the tastes of India with your guests and family. The uniqueness of the curry spice will create an exciting spice sensation to your palate. As you and your guests consume this curried creation, don't be surprised if they decide that a pilgrimage down the Ganges or a trip up Mt. Everest may be in order.

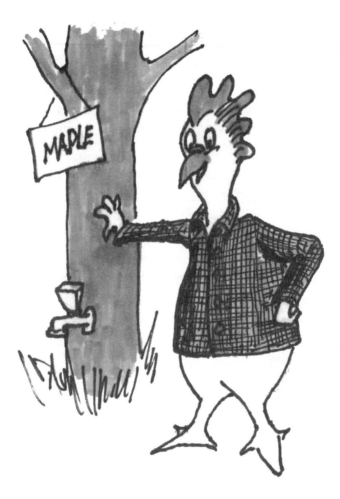

Zen and the Art of...

Vermont Maple Mudhen

The peaceful rolling countryside of Vermont with its dense forests of maple trees has been sited as the capitol of maple syrup. Tapping the maple and extracting the essence of the syrup has been practiced since before Ethan Allen wore diapers. The syrup's unique flavor and sweetness has blessed the pancakes of millions since. Taking a bold new step for this culinary icon of history and applying it to the continuous infusion process yields the Vermont Maple Mudhen. Yippee Skippee!

Vermont Maple Mudhen

Basic Stuff

1 3 to 6 lb. chicken
6 red potatoes
1 onion sliced
½ c. tarragon vinegar
½ c. maple syrup
¼ c. Dijon mustard
¼ c. vegetable or extra virgin olive oil

Rub

2 Tbs. garlic powder
1 Tbs. Kosher or Sea Salt
1 Tbs. black pepper

Liquid Flavor Essence

10 oz. dark beer
 4 oz. Canadian whiskey

Cooking Directions

➢ Mix the olive oil, vinegar, maple syrup, mustard and rub spices in a bowl, stirring to a smooth consistency.

➢ Using a basting brush, paint the critter with the glaze. Put some glaze aside for basting later.

➢ Add the liquid flavor essence to the flavor base of the cooker.

➢ Place the bird on the flavor tower.

➢ Line the base of the bird with the sliced onions and potatoes.

➢ Cover the chicken with a brown paper bag.

➢ In a conventional oven, cook at 325° for 1½ to 2 hours. In the last 20 minutes of cooking, remove the paper bag and baste the chicken. Cook until the drippings are clear and the leg quarters move easily in their joints.

➢ If grilling, follow the indirect heating method as explained on page 25.

Serve with a fresh salad, steamed zucchini strips and dinner rolls. Revel in the warmth of your home and the love of your people. Chop plenty of wood before you serve this delectable because you'll want to savor the bliss of this fine New England creation.

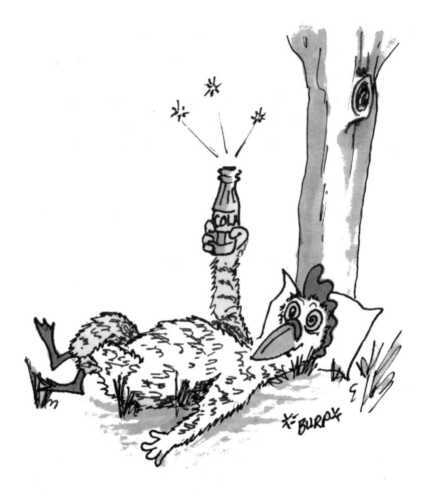

Zen and the Art of...

Carbonated Cola Cuckoo

Great cooks all over the world have often created dishes combining the zestiness of spice with the sweetness of sugar. This All-American classic is no exception. The sweetness of cola combined with the flavor of the chili pepper work together to create a concoction fit for a summer afternoon playing baseball and smelling the freshly mowed grass. Though this recipe calls for cola, other elixirs such as root beer, cherry cola or other soda pop flavor have been found to work wonderfully in combination with the spiciness of the rub. Zoom!

Carbonated Cola Cuckoo

Basic Stuff

1 3 to 6 lb. chicken
¼ c. vegetable or extra virgin olive oil

Rub

1 Tbs. Kosher or Sea Salt
1 Tbs. black pepper
2 Tbs. garlic powder
2 Tbs. chili powder
1 Tbs. ground cumin
1 tsp. cayenne pepper

Liquid Flavor Essence

16 oz. cola

Cooking Directions

➤ Make a glaze by whisking together the olive oil and ½ c cola.

➤ Using a basting brush, paint the critter with the glaze. Put some glaze aside for basting later.

➤ Add the cola to the flavor base of the cooker.

➤ Place the bird on the flavor tower.

➤ In a conventional oven, cook at 350° for 1½ hours. In the last 20 minutes of cooking, baste the chicken with some remaining glaze.

➤ Cook until the drippings are clear and the leg quarters move easily in their joints.

➤ If grilling, follow the indirect heating method as explained on page 25.

Serve with a potato salad, corn on the cob and baked beans. This tasty summer concoction will have everyone running out and doing somersaults in the grass while clucking with enthusiasm. Do not worry about such behavior as studies have shown it to be a healthy expression of gastric delight.

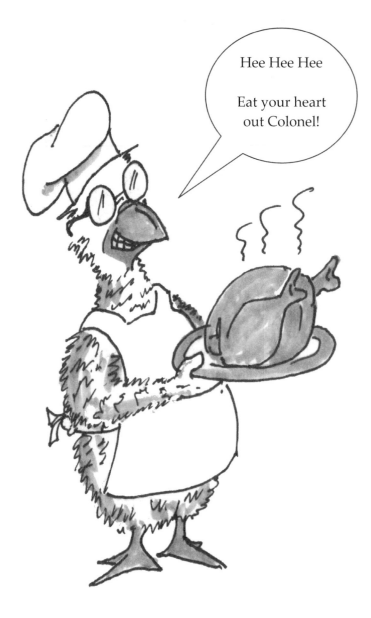

Donald's Delightful Dork Bird

This recipe, invented by the illustrator of this fine cookbook, demonstrates how simple approaches to culinary creations can yield incredible and serendipitous results. We don't need to have all the fancy-schmancy ingredients with multiple cooking steps and sauces prepared in advance. Sometimes it is good to take a step back, throw on a dab of this and dollop of that, kick back, chill and contemplate the Universe while gazing into the infinite spaces off our sundecks.

Donald's Delightful Dork Bird

Basic Stuff
1 3 to 6 lb. chicken
¼ c. vegetable or extra virgin olive oil

Rub
2 Tbs. garlic powder
2 Tbs. lemon pepper
1 Tbs. chili pepper
1 tsp. Kosher or Sea Salt
1 tsp. black pepper

Liquid Flavor Essence
32 oz. of the beer of your choice

Cooking Directions

➢ Using a basting brush, paint the critter with the olive oil.

➢ Apply the rub evenly over the bird.

➢ Add the 12 oz. of the beer to the flavor base.

➢ Place the bird on the flavor tower.

➢ In a conventional oven, cook at 350° for 1½ hours.

➢ Drink the remaining 20oz. of beer as the bird cooks.

➢ Cook until the drippings are clear and the leg quarters move easily in their joints.

➢ If grilling, follow the indirect heating method as explained on page 25.

Serve with a fresh salad, dilled green beans, baked potatoes and dinner rolls. Enjoy the simplicity and ease of this recipe preparation. This is definitely a bird to be enjoyed in a peaceful mental mode with no worries, sunshine and the giggles of small children.

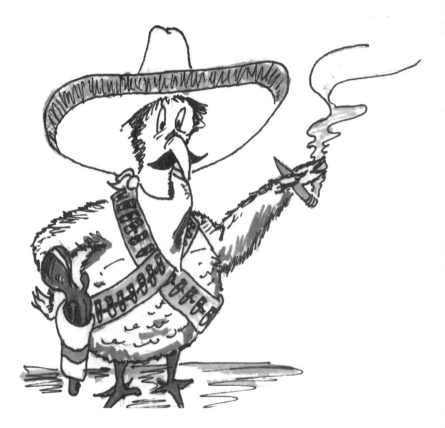

Chipotle Chicken Roast

There is nothing like the heat and elegance of slow smoked jalapeno peppers in adobo sauce. The heat essence of the jalapeno combined with the smokiness of the mesquite chip makes a wonderfully unique flavor. This recipe is reserved for those who enjoy and relish the culinary explosion of spice and heat. This bird is not for the faint of heart!

Chipotle Chicken Roast

Basic Stuff

1 3 to 6 lb. chicken
1 7oz. can of Chipotles in Adobo sauce
1 onion sliced
1 green pepper sliced

Rub

1 Tbs. garlic powder
1 Tbs. chili pepper
1 Tbs. cumin
1 tsp. cayenne pepper
1 tsp. Kosher or Sea Salt
1 tsp. black pepper

Liquid Flavor Essence

6 oz. dark beer
6 oz. Tequila

Cooking Directions

➤ Using a basting brush, paint the critter with the Adobo sauce from the can of Chipotles.

➤ Apply the rub evenly over the bird.

➤ Add liquid flavor essence to the flavor base.

➤ Place the bird on the flavor tower.

➤ Arrange the Chipotle peppers, onion slices and green pepper around the base of the bird.

➤ In a conventional oven, cook at 350° for 1½ hours.

➤ Cook until the drippings are clear and the leg quarters move easily in their joints.

➤ If grilling, follow the indirect heating method as explained on page 25.

Serve with a fresh fruit salad, corn on the cob, steamed peas, tortilla chips and corn bread. Have plenty of beverages available for this squawker as the spice and heat of the Chipotle will have your dinner guests reaching for their glasses. As such prepare yourself for many toasts and words of praise as the heat permeates the palates and good cheer fills the ambiance of your kitchen.

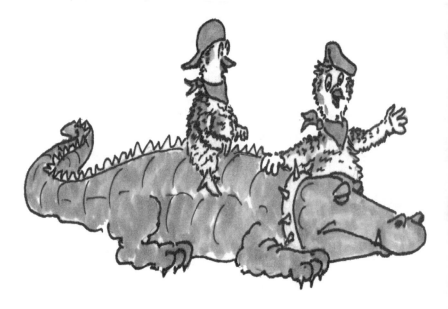

Zen and the Art of...

Cajun Blackened Chicken Roast

Wild spirit and fanciful culinary explosions come to the fore with the heat and flavor of a good blackened chicken. Served up with the spirit of New Orleans to sway your diners with the laid back ambiance and underlying wildness of Bourbon Street and those oh-so-sweet decadent memories of Mardi Gras.

Cajun Blackened Chicken Roast

Basic Stuff

1 3 to 6 lb. chicken
1 onion sliced
1 green pepper sliced
1 dozen sliced okra
½ c. olive oil

Rub

1 Tbs. garlic powder
1 Tbs. chili pepper
1 Tbs. cumin
1 tsp. cayenne pepper
1 tsp. Kosher or Sea Salt
1 tsp. black pepper

Liquid Flavor Essence

12 oz. dark beer

Cooking Directions

➤ Using a basting brush, paint the critter with the olive oil.

➤ Apply the rub evenly over the bird.

➤ Add liquid flavor essence to the flavor base.

➤ Place the bird on the flavor tower.

➤ Arrange the vegetables around the base of the bird.

➤ In a conventional oven, cook at 350° for 1½ hours.

➤ Cook until the drippings are clear and the leg quarters move easily in their joints.

➤ If grilling, follow the indirect heating method as explained on page 25.

Serve with jambalaya, a tossed salad, a side of smoked sausage, black beans with rice and finish up with some mint juleps. Let the Cajun spirit whisk you away into dreams of hot Louisiana summers, fine jazz and great food.

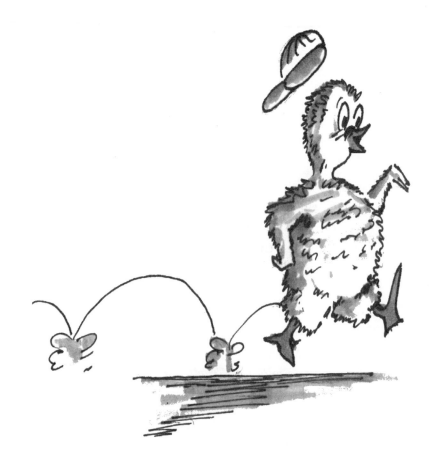

Kentucky Baseball Picnic Bird

Here's a chicken recipe straight out of Grandma's recipe book. This concoction captures the spirit of the old south with its warm days and the breezes of the Appalachian countryside whispering over fields of grass. Listen to the happy sounds of guitars and violins, stompin' out jigs and square dances as large groups of friends and family soak up the sun and enjoy warm summer picnics.

Kentucky Baseball Picnic Bird

Basic Stuff

1 3 to 6 lb. chicken
3-4 Tbs. Louisiana hot sauce
4 sliced apples
¼ cube butter

Rub

¼ c. fresh basil
1 Tbs. garlic powder
1 tsp. Kosher or Sea Salt
1 tsp. black pepper

Liquid Flavor Essence

8 oz. beer
½ c Southern Comfort

Cooking Directions

➢ Melt the butter and add the Louisiana Hot Sauce and paint the critter using a basting brush.

➢ Apply the rub evenly over the bird.

➢ Add liquid flavor essence to the flavor base.

➢ Place the bird on the flavor tower.

➢ Arrange the apple slices around the base of the bird.

➢ In a conventional oven, cook at 350° for 1½ hours.

➢ Cook until the drippings are clear and the leg quarters move easily in their joints.

➢ If grilling, follow the indirect heating method as explained on page 25.

Serve with a black-eyed pea salad, fresh bread rolls and baked potatoes. Be prepared to get caught up in the revelry of fun and sun, Rebel yells and foot-stompin' fun.

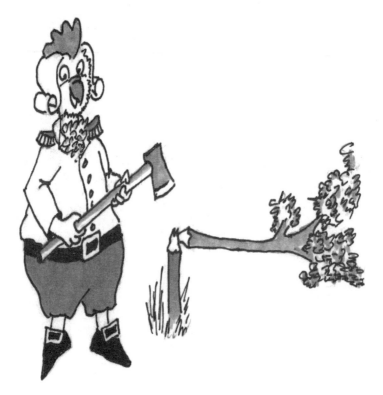

Zen and the Art of...

Traverse City Cherry Delight

On the northern Lower Peninsula of Michigan, Traverse City beckons lovers of sun, beaches, sailing and the festive taste of cherries. Indeed, Traverse City has become the Cherry Capital of the World. One can walk along the sidewalks of the downtown area and purchase everything from cherry sausage to cherry ice cream. It is appropriate that this cherry-flavor chicken concoction share its place at the tables of those cherry-loving, northern Michigan enthusiasts. George Washington would have thought twice about chopping a cherry tree down had he known of the sweet cherry chicken concoction contrived from the cherries.

Traverse City Cherry Delight

Basic Stuff
1 3 to 6 lb. chicken
3 finely chopped garlic cloves
1 onion chopped
4 oz. blush wine
½ lb. sliced black cherries
¼ lb. butter

Rub
1 Tbs. garlic powder
1 tsp. Kosher or Sea Salt
1 tsp. black pepper

Liquid Flavor Essence
6 oz. of cherry cola
4 oz. blush wine
4 oz. of brandy

Cooking Directions

➤ Sauté the cherries, garlic and onion in ¼ lb. butter and 4 oz. of the blush wine and set aside.

➤ Melt the remaining butter and paint the critter with a basting brush.

➤ Apply the rub evenly over the bird.

➤ Add liquid flavor essence to the flavor base.

➤ Place the bird on the flavor tower.

➤ Arrange the cherry, garlic and onion sauté around the base of the bird.

➤ In a conventional oven, cook at 350° for 1½ hours.

➤ Cook until the drippings are clear and the leg quarters move easily in their joints.

➤ If grilling, follow the indirect heating method as explained on page 25.

Serve with a fresh fruit salad, corn on the cob, dilled asparagus, mashed potatoes and sourdough bread. Ladle portions of the baked cherry sauté over the spuds. Enjoy the sweetness and spirit of the North mingling with hot beaches and warm sun. Get your golf clubs, rent a ski boat or just kick back.

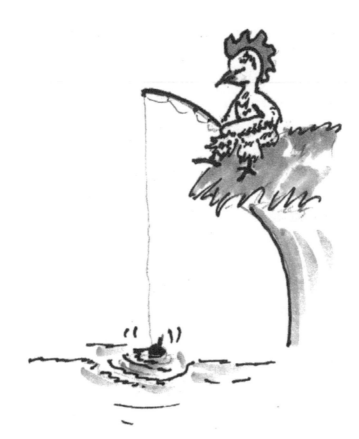

Zen and the Art of...

Hollingsworth's Hellacious Swimming Hen

A Michigan outdoor enthusiast and avid salmon fisherman was enjoying the cool morning while standing in his waders in a fast moving stream in Northern Michigan.

His thoughts drifted to how good that salmon would taste with that special marinade of his own invention. As he patiently waited for that familiar tug on his fishing pole, his mouth began to water in anticipation.

Suddenly, his fishing line went taught...he had snagged a beauty; full of fight and spirit. He reeled the twisting and fighting catch in. Finally, with a splash, he pulled it out of the water and saw he had snagged a rare Northern Michigan swimming chicken.

His hunger and desire for a truly fine meal overcame his fishing sensibilities, so he trundled off to camp. The meal he came up with became famous in Northern Michigan as Hollingsworth's Hellacious Swimming Hen. The rest is history.

Hollingsworth's Hellacious Swimming Hen

Basic Stuff

1 3 to 6 lb. chicken
3 finely chopped garlic cloves
1 onion chopped
¼ lb. butter
½ c. red wine
½ c. olive oil

Rub

2 Tbs. garlic powder
1 Tbs. dill weed
1 tsp. Kosher or Sea Salt
1 tsp. black pepper

Liquid Flavor Essence

6 oz. red wine
6 oz. cherry-lime soda

Cooking Directions

➤ Sauté the garlic and onion in ¼ lb. butter and ½ cup of the red wine and set aside.

➤ Apply the olive oil over the bird.

➤ Apply the rub evenly over the bird.

➤ Add liquid flavor essence to the flavor base.

➤ Stuff the sautéed garlic and onion into the neck cavity of the bird.

➤ Place the bird on the flavor tower.

➤ In a conventional oven, cook at 350° for 1½ hours.

➤ Cook until the drippings are clear and the leg quarters move easily in their joints.

➤ If grilling, follow the indirect heating method as explained on page 25.

Serve with a fresh salad garden salad with artichoke hearts, steamed red potatoes, merlot-sautéed portabella mushrooms (page 182) and fresh French bread. Sit back, enjoy the meal and discuss the merits of fishing and communing with the Great Outdoors. Drink toasts to your friends and engage in lively debates regarding social welfare, politic and the Zen qualities of the Hellacious Hen.

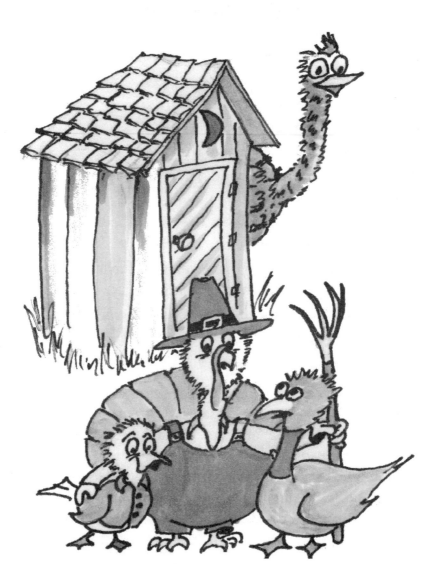

Zen and the Art of...

The Delightful Digression of An Infused Turkey

As you have figured out by now, chickens cooked using the continuous infusion process are tender, flavor and fun to cook. This section expands the use of "beer-can" poultry to include turkey.

The continuous infusion process generates the same effect observed with using chickens. The liquid flavor base imparts flavor steam inside the critter, while the outside heat of the grill or oven crisp up the skin locking and loading the moisture and juices inside.

It is no different with turkeys and other critters. Indeed, a 12 to 20 lb. turkey will cook up nicely. Allow roughly 10 to 12 minutes per pound. For turkey, it is a good idea to use a secondary pan to set the cooker in to catch any possible overflow during cooking.

Note that turkeys cook best when placed neck down on the tower of an infusion cooker. Obviously using an infusion cooker is preferable as actual beer-cans are not stable, particularly for larger poultry.

Make sure that if you are doing a bigger bird that you make sure it will fir in your oven or grill. The tail can be trimmed down to accommodate it if the bird is too tall.

If actually using a beer-can for your turkey, place the turkey butt-down. You may need to carve the tail end of the bird to assist it in standing up right as the turkeys tend to be top-heavy. You may also need to provide additional stability for the turkey, while she's cooking. She can be propped up using three pre-cleaned rocks arranged around the bird in a triangular fashion as a support.

Actual beer-cans are not recommended for turkeys as the birds are so much bigger then conventional chickens; however, it is possible with a little care and proper preparation.

You can actually stuff the bird because its butt will be stickin' up.

Try some of these recipes and enjoy the expanded versatility of continuous infusion cooking.

Try any of the brining or injectable approaches with your continuously infused turkey.

Check out our video at: **redowlpubblications.com.**

Traditional Turkey

Basic Stuff

1 10 to 20 lb. thawed turkey
8 red potatoes
1 onion chopped
¼ c. olive oil
¼ lb. butter

Rub

2 Tbs. garlic powder
1 Tbs. rosemary
1 Tbs. sage
1 tsp. Kosher or Sea Salt
1 tsp. black pepper

Liquid Flavor Essence

18 oz. highly hopped beer
4 oz. cranberry juice

Cooking Directions

➤ Remove giblets and wash out inside of bird.

➤ Place your turkey neck down on your infusion cooker. The other end is a bit too large and the bird's center of gravity will work against you if you stick it down butt first.

➤ Pat the bird dry with paper towels and apply olive oil over the outside of the turkey.

➤ Apply the rub evenly over the bird.

➤ Add liquid flavor essence to the flavor base.

➤ Place the bird on the flavor tower.

➤ Arrange the chopped onion and potatoes around the bird in the flavor base.

➤ Always use a secondary pan to set the chicken cooker in as there is a potential for overflow.

➤ Make sure the bird fits in your oven or grill. If neck down, the butt end can be trimmed to fit if necessary.

➤ In a conventional oven, cook at 350° allowing about 12 minutes per pound, or cook until the inside thigh temperature is 180 ° F.

➤ Cook until the drippings are clear and the leg quarters move easily in their joints.

➤ If grilling, follow the indirect heating method as explained on page 25.

Serve with all the traditional side dishes associated with Thanksgiving and slow cooked turkey and enjoy the Zen peace of a tender juicy turkey gracing your table.

Cajun Gobbler

Basic Stuff

1 10 to 20 lb. turkey
1 onion sliced
1 green pepper sliced
1 dozen sliced okra
½ c. olive oil

Rub

1 Tbs. garlic powder
1 Tbs. chili powder
1 Tbs. cumin
1 tsp. cayenne pepper
1 tsp. Kosher or Sea Salt
1 tsp. black pepper

Liquid Flavor Essence

24 oz. dark beer

Cooking Directions

➤ Remove giblets and wash out inside of bird.

➤ Place your turkey neck down on your infusion cooker. The other end is a bit too large and the bird's center of gravity will work against you if you stick it down butt first.

➤ For extra Cajun appeal try recipe with the Cluckin Cajun Cuckoo Bird Brine (page 42), or inject with the Cajun Creole Injectable Delight (page 47), varying the cook time appropriately.

➤ Pat the bird dry with paper towels and apply olive oil over the outside of the turkey.

➤ Apply the rub evenly over the bird.

➤ Add liquid flavor essence to the flavor base.

➤ Place the bird on the flavor tower.

➤ Arrange the vegetables around the base of the bird.

➤ Always use a secondary pan to set the chicken cooker in as there is a potential for overflow.

➤ Make sure the bird fits in your oven or grill. If neck down, the butt end can be trimmed to fit if necessary.

➤ In a conventional oven, cook at 350° allowing about 12 minutes per pound, or cook until the inside thigh temperature is 180 ° F.

➤ Cook until the drippings are clear and the leg quarters move easily in their joints.

➤ If grilling, follow the indirect heating method as explained on page 25.

Serve with jambalaya, a tossed salad, a side of fresh peas and baby corn with dill (page 174) and finish up with some mint juleps. Kick back and listen to the early evening sounds of the Bayou...and contemplate the Zen of the Cajun Gobbler!

Transylvanian Turkey

Basic Stuff
1 10 to 20 lb. thawed turkey
¼ c. olive oil

Rub
2 Tbs. garlic powder
1 Tbs. basil
1 Tbs. dill weed
1 tsp. Kosher or Sea Salt
1 tsp. black pepper

Liquid Flavor Essence
12 oz. Chardonnay wine
8 oz. cranberry juice

Cooking Directions

➤ Remove giblets and wash out inside of bird.

➤ Place your turkey neck down on your infusion cooker. The other end is a bit too large and the bird's center of gravity will work against you if you stick it down butt first.

➤ For extra appeal try recipe injecting with Czar Nick's Injection Sauce (page 49).

➤ Pat the bird dry with paper towels and apply olive oil over the outside of the turkey.

➤ Apply the rub evenly over the bird.

➤ Add liquid flavor essence to the flavor base.

➤ Place the bird on the flavor tower.

➤ Always use a secondary pan to set the chicken cooker in as there is a potential for overflow.

➤ Make sure the bird fits in your oven or grill. If neck down, the butt end can be trimmed to fit if necessary.

➤ In a conventional oven, cook at 350° allowing about 12 minutes per pound, or cook until the inside thigh temperature is 180 ° F.

➤ Cook until the drippings are clear and the leg quarters move easily in their joints.

➤ If grilling, follow the indirect heating method as explained on page 25.

Serve with mashed potatoes and gravy, a Nutty Asparagus Salad (page 180), a side of fresh peas, and finish up with some lively toasts of a dry red vintage (with enthusiasm and Zen peace). Count Vlad would have been proud at this nifty concoction.

Shanghai Travelin' Turkey

Basic Stuff

1 10 to 20 lb. thawed turkey
Awesome Asian Bird Brine (page 41)
¼ c. olive oil and soy sauce, mixed 50-50

Rub

1 c. finely chopped peanuts
2 Tbs. garlic powder
1 Tbs. grated lemon peel
1 tsp. black pepper

Liquid Flavor Essence

4 oz. Teriyaki Sauce
18 oz. Sapporo Beer

Cooking Directions

➤ Remove giblets and wash out inside of bird.

➤ Place your turkey neck down on your infusion cooker. The other end is a bit too large and the bird's center of gravity will work against you if you stick it down butt first.

➤ Follow the brining instructions on page 40.

➤ Pat the bird dry with paper towels and apply olive oil/soy sauce mixture over the outside of the turkey.

➤ Apply the rub evenly over the bird.

➤ Add liquid flavor essence to the flavor base.

➤ Place the bird on the flavor tower.

➤ Always use a secondary pan to set the chicken cooker in as there is a potential for overflow.

➤ Make sure the bird fits in your oven or grill. If neck down, the butt end can be trimmed to fit if necessary.

➤ In a conventional oven, cook at 350° allowing about 8 minutes per pound (if brined) or 12 minutes per pound (if not brined), or cook until the inside thigh temperature is 180 ° F.

➤ Cook until the drippings are clear and the leg quarters move easily in their joints.

➤ If grilling, follow the indirect heating method as explained on page 25.

Serve with rice and stir-fried veggies, flavored with Peking Peanut Sauce (page 37).

Enjoy the subtle tastes of this buzzard in the comfort and safety of your home…no worries about being whisked off to serve time on the open seas…Just some peace, some Zen, some creative culinary excellence for your family and friends…

Turkey Milano

Basic Stuff
1 10 to 20 lb. turkey
½ c. olive oil

Rub
½ c. grated Parmesan cheese
1 Tbs. garlic powder
1 Tbs. basil
1 Tbs. onion powder
1 tsp. oregano
1 tsp. Kosher or Sea Salt

Liquid Flavor Essence
18 oz. Shiraz

Cooking Directions

➤ Remove giblets and wash out inside of bird.

➤ Place your turkey neck down on your infusion cooker. The other end is a bit too large and the bird's center of gravity will work against you if you stick it down butt first.

➤ Pat the bird dry with paper towels and apply olive oil over the outside of the turkey.

➤ Apply the rub evenly over the bird.

➤ Add liquid flavor essence to the flavor base.

➤ Place the bird on the flavor tower.

➤ Always use a secondary pan to set the chicken cooker in as there is a potential for overflow.

➤ Make sure the bird fits in your oven or grill. If neck down, the butt end can be trimmed to fit if necessary.

➤ In a conventional oven, cook at 350° allowing about 12 minutes per pound, or cook until the inside thigh temperature is 180 ° F.

➤ Cook until the drippings are clear and the leg quarters move easily in their joints.

➤ If grilling, follow the indirect heating method as explained on page 25.

➤

➤ Serve with Alfredo noodles, roasted corn on the cob (cooked on the grill!) and lightly glazed carrots.

➤

➤ Catch the essence of the Italian countryside as you imbibe this delectable…enjoy and Bang-Zoom!

Angi's Angelic Turkey Delight

Basic Stuff
1 10 to 20 lb. turkey
1 onion sliced
½ c. olive oil

Rub
1 Tbs. sage
1 Tbs. celery salt
1 Tbs. garlic powder
1 Tbs. onion powder
1 tsp. Kosher or Sea Salt
1 tsp. black pepper

Liquid Flavor Essence
24 oz. your favorite stout beer

Cooking Directions

➤ Remove giblets and wash out inside of bird.

➤ Place your turkey neck down on your infusion cooker. The other end is a bit too large and the bird's center of gravity will work against you if you stick it down butt first.

➤ Pat the bird dry with paper towels and apply olive oil over the outside of the turkey.

➤ Apply the rub evenly over the bird.

➤ Add liquid flavor essence to the flavor base. Add the onion and giblets to the flavor base.

➤ Place the bird on the flavor tower.

➤ Always use a secondary pan to set the chicken cooker in as there is a potential for overflow.

➤ Make sure the bird fits in your oven or grill. If neck down, the butt end can be trimmed to fit if necessary.

➤ In a conventional oven, cook at 350° allowing about 12 minutes per pound, or cook until the inside thigh temperature is 180 ° F.

➤ Cook until the drippings are clear and the leg quarters move easily in their joints.

➤ If grilling, follow the indirect heating method as explained on page 25.

➤ Save the used liquid flavor essence and make genuine giblet gravy.

Serve with sage stuffing, biscuits and giblet gravy, and fresh dark salad greens with light rice vinegar and oil dressing.

Enjoy and rock and roll with this delicious variation on the traditional Thanksgiving theme!

Assorted Appetizers, Accompaniments and Anecdotal Aphorisms

Creation by cooking has always been a favored form of human expression. The previous chicken and turkey recipes capture but a fraction of the infinite possibilities. A dab of this, a splash of that: all joining together in a symphony of culinary splendor.

The uniqueness of the continuous infusion poultry cooking is that such an approach allows for a tremendous amount of creativity. One would have to put forth a concerted effort to make a bird that tasted bad using a continuous infusion cooker. Thus, with the cooker itself nearly assuring success, creative license is thrust wide open. Whatever tastes good to you can be creatively applied to a unique and exciting recipe using this approach to cooking chicken.

The following are tried and true recipes, which have been noted to compliment the chicken recipes previously presented.

Enjoy and Bon Appétit!

Ricotta Stuffed Portabella Mushrooms

Basic Stuff

4-6 large whole Portabella mushroom caps
2 c. ricotta cheese
1 c. cream cheese
½ c. grated Parmesan cheese
½ c. capers
¼ c. brandy
2 Tbs. garlic powder
2 Tbs. basil

Cooking Directions

Mix the ricotta, cream cheese, capers, brandy and spices. Fill each mushroom cap with the mixture. Place on a cookie sheet and bake for 45 minutes at 350°. Remove from oven and sprinkle the Parmesan cheese over the tops.

Alternatively, the stuffed mushrooms can be placed around the base of the chicken and cooked with the delightful bird. This delicacy will certainly add a bit pizzazz to your extraordinary meal.

Fresh Asparagus with Dill Sauce

Basic Stuff
2 lb. fresh steamed asparagus

Sauce
3 minced garlic cloves
1 c. plain yogurt
½ c cream
2 Tbs. minced dill
½ tsp. salt

Cooking Directions

In a saucepan over gentle heat, combine the sauce ingredients. Stir continuously to mix and prevent scalding.

Ladle desired sauce quantity over individual asparagus servings and enjoy.

Fresh Peas and Baby Corn with Dill

Basic Stuff
1 lb. frozen peas
1 can baby corn

Sauce
3 minced garlic cloves
1 c. plain yogurt
½ c. cream
2 Tbs. minced dill
½ tsp. salt

Cooking Directions

Cut the baby corn into 1" segments and cook with the frozen peas. Add a dollop of butter to the mix prior to serving.

In a saucepan over gentle heat, combine the sauce ingredients. Stir continuously to mix and prevent scalding.

Ladle desired sauce quantity over vegetable servings and enjoy, while you explore profound philosophical concepts through engaging conversation.

Coconut Shrimp

Basic Stuff

1 lb. large shelled shrimp
3 c. vegetable oil
1 c. shredded coconut

Batter

1 egg
1 c. cream
½ c. brown sugar
½ c. all-purpose flour
½ Tbs. garlic powder
1 tsp. chopped cilantro
½ tsp. crushed red chili pepper

Cooking Directions

Prepare the batter by adding the egg, spices, cream and sugar. While mixing, gradually add the flour to allow for even mixing until the batter is smooth in consistency.

Place the shredded coconut in a separate bowl. Dip the shrimp in the batter mix and then roll in the coconut until completely covered.

Fry the coated shrimps in the oil until golden brown in color.

This beauty of a dish makes for a great appetizer or fine accompaniment to any of your cooking efforts.

Stuffed Spiced Zucchini

Basic Stuff

2 large zucchini
1 chopped onion
1 egg
1 c. Romano cheese
1 c. scrambled breakfast sausage
1 c. steamed rice
1 c. mozzarella cheese
¼ c. virgin olive oil
2 Tbs. garlic powder
2 Tbs. crushed and chopped basil
1 tsp. red pepper

Cooking Directions

Cut zucchini in half lengthwise. Scoop out the seeds. Scoop out the meat and put aside. Boil the zucchini until they are soft and tender. Mix the rice, onion, Romano cheese, egg and spices with the zucchini meat. Fry the mixture in the olive oil for 3 to 4 minutes. Let stand. Stuff mixture into the zucchini, top with the mozzarella and bake at 300° for about an hour.

Black-Eyed Pea Salad

Basic Stuff

4 chopped garlic cloves
6 slices fried bacon
1 chopped red pepper
10 c. water
4 c. dried black-eyed peas
¼ c. dried cilantro
¼ c. chopped green onions
2 Tbs. curry powder
1 Tbs. salt
1 Tbs. garlic powder
½ tsp. chili powder
½ tsp. cumin

Dressing

½ c. red wine vinegar
½ c. virgin olive oil
¼ c. mayonnaise

Cooking Directions

Soak the peas with a ½ handful of salt over night. Drain, rinse and add the 10 cups of water. Bring to boiling and let simmer for 15 minutes. Drain and cool with cold water. Combine all the rest of the basic stuff and the dressing. Gently mix well and rock and roll with an awesome and unique salad experience.

Tequila Shrimp

Basic Stuff

4 finely chopped garlic cloves
1 coarsely chopped onion
1 coarsely chopped green pepper
3 coarsely chopped carrots
1 lb. unpeeled large shrimp
2 c. steamed rice
½ c. olive oil
½ c. tequila
¼ c. heavy whipping cream
¼ c. squeezed lime juice
2 Tbs. dried crushed red pepper
2 Tbs. vinegar

Cooking Directions

Peel shrimp, put in a baking pan with the vegetables and set aside. Combine the olive oil, tequila, lime juice, chopped garlic and red pepper and mix well. Add the vegetables to the shrimp. Marinate for an hour. Remove shrimp and vegetables and bring the remaining marinade to a boil then set aside. In a clean baking pan, lay the rice so as to form a layer on the bottom. Lay the shrimp and vegetables over the rice. Add the heavy cream over the cooled marinade and pour over the shrimp, vegetables and rice. Bake at 325° for about an hour or until the contents start to brown.

Coconut Rice

Basic Stuff

2 chopped onions
3 c. steamed rice
2½ c. water
½ cube butter
½ c. shredded coconut
½ c. heavy cream
1 Tbs. finely chopped ginger root
1 Tbs. Kosher or Sea Salt
1 Tbs. garlic powder
1 tsp. black pepper

Cooking Directions

In a saucepan, melt the butter and add the coconut, ginger, onions and spices. Add the rice, water and cream. Bring to a boil, cover and lightly simmer for about twenty minutes until the rice is done. A splash of teriyaki prior top serving is an option. Enjoy with any of the Asian-mode chicken recipes in this book (or any other for that matter). Be careful not to start dancing vigorously while preparing this dish. The cooking aromas may entice you but showing restraint is a measure of good quality in a human.

Nutty Asparagus Salad

Basic Stuff

1 dozen spears of asparagus
3 c. small cooked spiral pasta
½ c. finely chopped red onion
½ c. halved cherry tomatoes
½ c. olive oil
3 Tbs. pine nuts
3 Tbs. slivered almonds
2 Tbs. Tarragon vinegar
1 Tbs. fresh horseradish
1 tsp. garlic powder
1 tsp. dill weed
½ tsp. lemon pepper

Cooking Directions

Cut the asparagus spears into 1½" segments. Blanch the asparagus spears until they are crisp yet tender (about 2 minutes). Drain. In a bowl combine the vinegar, horseradish, spices and olive oil. Whisk until smooth. Add the pasta followed by the vegetables and nuts. Toss gently to coat. Chill the mixture for about an hour prior to serving.

Baby Corn and Garlic Sauté

Basic Stuff

1 can baby corn
1 finely chopped red pepper
4 finely chopped garlic cloves
1 finely chopped small onion
½ c. chopped mushrooms
¼ c. white wine
1 tsp. lemon pepper
¼ lb. butter

Cooking Directions

Chop each baby corncob in half. Add the corn, garlic, onion, pepper, mushrooms and spices to a skillet and sauté in the butter until the onion starts to brown. Add the wine, cover and let simmer for about 3 minutes. Serve over rice or pasta.

Merlot-Sautéed Portabella Mushrooms

Basic Stuff

4 to 6 large, sectioned Portabella mushrooms
1 chopped onion
2 c. dry Merlot wine
¼ c. olive oil
2 Tbs. garlic powder
2 Tbs. crushed basil
1 tsp. oregano
1 tsp. salt
1 tsp. black pepper

Cooking Directions

In a frying pan, sauté the mushrooms, onion and spices in the olive oil until onion is slightly browned. Pour the Merlot over the mixture and cover and let simmer 5 minutes. This little creation is a great compliment, served over steak, chicken, fish, pasta or rice. It's simple, quick, elegant and tasty.

Baked Cheese Vegetable Medley

Basic Stuff

1 chopped onion
4 finely chopped garlic cloves
12 oz. shredded Colby-Jack cheese
1 can Cream of Mushroom soup
2 c. diced green beans
2 c. broccoli caps
2 c. yellow corn
2 c. mushrooms
2 c. water
1 c. dry rice
2 c. Potato cubes
½ c. dry white wine
¼ c. chopped carrots
2 Tbs. garlic powder
2 Tbs. black pepper

Cooking Directions

Add all the ingredients to a sufficiently large casserole dish, being sure to mix all the ingredients thoroughly. Bake at 350° for an hour. This vegetable delight will tickle the fancy of even the most stubborn vegetable eaters. It makes a great companion to any main course and is a great leftover when the party is over and the guests have left for their respective destinations.

Garlic Mushroom Ragout

Basic Stuff

1 lb. fresh mushrooms, sliced
1 10 oz. can of diced tomatoes, undrained
8 thinly sliced shallots
4 finely chopped garlic cloves
½ c. dry white wine
½ c. Romano cheese
3 Tbs. chopped parsley
2 Tbs. lemon juice
½ tsp. Kosher or Sea Salt
½ tsp. black pepper
¼ lb. butter, cut in small pieces

Cooking Directions

In a large bowl, mix mushrooms with shallots, garlic,
parsley, lemon juice, salt and pepper. In a deep frying pan,
sauté the mixture in the butter until tender, yet still firm.
Add the tomatoes and wine, cover and simmer for 10
minutes. Serve over meat, chicken, fish, pasta, rice or add
to a fresh tossed salad. Sprinkle the Romano cheese over
each serving and garnish with chopped parsley. Your
dinner guests will positively devour this embellishing
creation.

Brocolli Bacon Salad

Basic Stuff

1 large bunch broccoli, separated into florets
1 coarsely chopped large onion
10 to 12 bacon strips, cooked and crumbled
1 c. raisins
1 c. pine nuts
2 tsp. garlic powder
3¼ pinch Kosher or Sea Salt

Dressing

3 Tbs. vinegar
½ c. mayonnaise
½ c. brown sugar
¼ c. Dijon mustard

Cooking Directions

In a large bowl, mix up the broccoli, onion, raisins, pine nuts, garlic powder, salt and bacon; set aside. In another bowl, combine dressing ingredients. Before serving, pour dressing over the broccoli salad and toss. Make sure there are no rabbits nearby as they have been known to go into a rabbit frenzy whenever they smell this creative culinary creation.

Creole Black Beans and Rice

Basic Stuff

2 coarsely peeled and chopped tomatoes
1 finely chopped medium sized onion
3 finely chopped garlic cloves
1 chopped green pepper
½ dozen sectioned okra
3 c. cooked black beans
2 c. cold water
1½ c. uncooked rice
½ c. red wine
½ c. olive oil
2 tsp. black pepper
2 tsp. dried cayenne pepper
2 tsp. chili powder

Cooking Directions

Sauté the onion, garlic and pepper in olive oil until the onion is tender. Add the tomatoes and cook, stirring well until the mixture is well blended and thick. Season with salt and pepper to taste. Stir in the black beans and mix well. Add the rice, water and wine. Cover and simmer on low until rice is done and the moisture has been absorbed. Be aware that your guests may start singing jazz tunes and calling for crawfish heads…but don't worry, such episodes have been shown to be temporary.

Sea Critter Seasoned Fettuccine

Basic Stuff

8 oz. Fettuccine noodles
½ lb. smoked salmon
1 c. half-n-half
1 c. heavy cream
½ lb. peeled large shrimp
½ c. Irish whiskey
½ c. grated Parmesan cheese
¼ c. sea scallops
¼ c. mussels
¼ cube butter
¼ c. ricotta cheese
2 Tbs. chopped fresh parsley
1 Tbs. garlic powder
1 Tbs. dried basil
3 tsp. minced garlic
2 tsp. black pepper
1 tsp. Kosher or Sea Salt

Cooking Directions

Place the Fettuccine noodles, half-n-half, heavy cream, garlic and seafood in a saucepan and simmer under medium heat stirring continuously. Add the whiskey, butter, Ricotta cheese, spices; continue to simmer; stir until the mixture becomes thick. Pour onto a serving platter, sprinkle the top with Parmesan cheese and garnish with parsley prior to serving.

Curried Pasta Salad

Basic Stuff

12 oz. cooked and drained spiral pasta
1 apple, peeled and chopped
2 shredded carrots
¼ c. raisins
¼ c. green onion sliced into small rings
1 Tbs. mayonnaise or plain yogurt
1 Tbs. lemon juice
1 tsp. curry powder
1 tsp. garlic powder
1 tsp. teriyaki sauce

Cooking Directions

Mix spices, teriyaki sauce, mayonnaise and lemon juice into a dressing. Mix all the rest of the ingredients and serve chilled with sourdough bread. This salad is a fine accompaniment for the Indian and Asian recipes in this book

Parmesan Artichoke Ragout

Basic Stuff

1 14 oz. can diced tomatoes, undrained
1 10 oz. package frozen artichoke hearts
4 finely chopped garlic cloves
1 c. coarsely chopped green pepper
1 c. chopped onion
1 c. freshly grated Parmesan
1 c. dry red wine
1 c. chopped pitted olives
½ c. fresh peas
3 Tbs. olive oil

Cooking Directions

Heat the oil over moderately low heat; add the onion, bell pepper and garlic. Cook until softened. Add all the remaining ingredients, cover and simmer for 10 minutes or until slightly thickened. Serve over warm rice or pasta. Cover serving with more Parmesan cheese and garnish with chopped fresh parsley.

Eggplant Parmigiana

Basic Stuff

1 lb. fresh sliced mozzarella cheese
2 large eggplants
1 tsp. Kosher or Sea Salt
2 tsp. garlic powder
2 tsp. black
2 c. basic tomato sauce
1 c. chopped fresh basil
½ c. red wine
½ c. freshly grated Parmesan cheese
½ c. garlic crouton crumbs
¼ c. olive oil

Cooking directions

Slice each eggplant into 6 pieces about 1" thick and soak in saltwater for 30 minutes prior to cooking. Season each disk with salt, pepper and garlic powder and place on the olive-oiled sheet. Bake the eggplant at 450° until the slices begin turning deep brown on top, about 15 minutes, remove and cool. Lower the oven temperature to 350°. In an 8" x 12" baking pan, place four of the eggplant slices evenly spaced apart. Spread some tomato sauce and basil over each slice. Place one slice of mozzarella over each and sprinkle with 1 tsp. grated Parmesan cheese. Layer the slices of eggplant and continuously repeat with tomato sauce, basil and the 2 cheeses. Sprinkle the crouton crumbs over the top of the eggplant dish and bake uncovered for 20 minutes or until the cheese melts and the tops turn light brown.

Seafood Gazpacho

Basic Stuff

1 large peeled and coarsely chopped cucumber
1 chopped onion
1 chopped green pepper
4 finely chopped garlic cloves
4 bay leaves
1-14 oz. can diced tomatoes, undrained
2 c. spicy V-8 juice
1½ c. water
1 c. white wine
¼ c. tarragon vinegar
½ lb. unpeeled large shrimp
½ lb. bay scallops
¼ lb. mussels
¼ lb. shredded cooked crab
2 Tbs. sugar
½ tsp. Kosher or Sea Salt
½ tsp. black pepper
½ tsp. oregano

Cooking Directions

The night before you desire to serve this delectable delight, add the cucumber, green pepper, onion and garlic to a food processor and puree until smooth. Add the remaining ingredients and mix well. Cover and chill overnight. 20 minutes prior serving, bring the water and wine to a boil and add peeled shrimp, scallops and mussels and cook 5 minutes. Drain and add crab, then chill. Immediately before serving, add the seafood to the Gazpacho base. This cold soup is a hearty accompaniment to any main course.

Feel free to add some zest with some hot pepper sauce and/or a dash cayenne pepper.

Zesty Zucchini Side Dish

Basic Stuff
1 medium zucchini sliced
2 medium garden tomatoes sliced
1 thinly sliced sweet onion
1 c. freshly grated Parmesan cheese
1 c. Italian seasoned breadcrumbs
¼ c. olive oil
¼ lb. butter

Cooking Directions
Coat an 8" square pan with the olive oil. Place zucchini slices (about ¼ " thick) on the bottom. Add a layer of thinly sliced onion, then a layer of tomato slices. Top that with the cheese. Add another layer of each vegetable, more cheese and top with breadcrumbs. Some finely chopped fresh basil mixed throughout is very tasty. Place a few dollops of butter atop the breadcrumbs. Bake uncovered at 350° for about 45 minutes. Use this recipe is to finish up all those garden zucchinis and tomatoes. A great accompaniment to infusion-cooked poultry!

Homestyle Bird 'n Noodle Soup

You've done it! You have infusion cooked your bird and satisfied the palettes of your family and guests. For clean-up turn all that is leftover into fine poultry soup that will stick to the ribs of your diners for days yet to come.

Basic Stuff

1 c. pasta noodles
1 c. white rice
¼ c. olive oil
¼ c. white wine
¼ c. sliced celery
Left-over chicken or turkey carcass
6 peeled and chopped cloves of garlic
1 medium chopped onion
¼ lb. baby carrots
¼ lb. diced green beans
¼ lb. fresh peas
1 Tbs. Kosher or Sea salt

Cooking Directions

Boil your leftover bird carcass in enough salted water to cover it for about 20 minutes. Using a strainer, drain the broth and save. Remove all the extra meat and add to the broth. Discard the bird bones. Bring broth and meat to a boil. Reduce heat to low, add the rest of the ingredients and allow soup to simmer for 30 to 45 minutes.

Serve with a tossed salad and some fresh dinner rolls.

Hoohaw Delight and Delicious Desserts

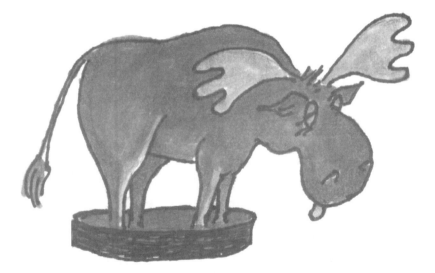

Wicked Chocolate Mousse

Basic Stuff

1 lb. finely chopped semisweet chocolate
1 lb. softened cream cheese
1 c. heavy cream
¼ c. slivered almonds
½ c. Brandy and Benedictine (B & B)

Cooking Directions

Melt the chocolate. In a bowl mix the cream and the cream cheese until smooth. Stir in the chocolate, almonds and the B&B. The consistency can be adjusted by adding more cream cheese for thickening or more cream for thinning. Spoon into individual pudding bowls and garnish with a dollop of whipped cream and a mint sprig. This creation makes for a nice conclusion to a fine meal. Bon Appétit!

Blarney Cheesecake

Basic Stuff

2 lbs. softened cream cheese
¼ lb. butter
8 oz. Graham cracker crumbs
6 eggs
1 Tbs. vanilla extract
2 c. sour cream
1 c. sugar
½ c. Bailey's Irish Cream

Cooking Directions

In a mixing bowl, whip the cream cheese and sugar until
well mixed. Continue beating and gradually add the eggs
followed by the vanilla and Irish Cream. Scrape the bowl
down several times during the mixing process. Prepare a 9"
spring-form pan by greasing with butter. Coat the inside of
the pan with a thin layer of the Graham cracker crumbs.
Pour the filling into the pan and bake at 325° for about an
hour or until filling is set and the edges begin cracking.
Allow the cake to cool and top with whipped cream prior to
serving.

Sweet Georgia Roasted Peaches

Basic Stuff

4 firm, ripe peaches
4 c. brown sugar
¼ lb. butter
1 c. heavy cream
2 Tbs. brandy
1 tsp. vanilla extract

Cooking Directions

Slice the peaches in halves and remove pits; place peaches
on cookie sheet. Place a dollop of butter in the holes and
pack full with brown sugar. Broil on high until brown
sugar starts to melt and bubble (about 10 minutes).
Remove from the oven and allow to cool. Combine the
heavy cream, vanilla and brandy into a bowl and whip until
thick. Top the peaches with whipped cream and serve.

Decadent Multi-Chocolated Cookies

Basic Stuff

4 squares semi-sweet chocolate
1 beaten egg
2 c. graham cracker crumbs
2 c. powdered sugar
1 c. coconut
1 c. chopped walnuts
½ c. powdered sugar
1 c. butter
1 Tbs. cocoa
3 Tbs. milk
1 tsp. vanilla
2 Tbs. instant vanilla pudding

Cooking Directions

Stir ½ c. of butter, the powdered sugar, the cocoa, the vanilla and the egg over low heat until well blended. Mix the graham cracker crumbs, coconut and walnuts into blended mixture. Pat the mixture into a 9" x 13" pan. In a separate pan, heat ½ c. butter, the milk, the powdered sugar, and the instant vanilla pudding until blended, then spread over the first mixture in the pan. Let stand 15 minutes. Finally, melt 4 squares chocolate with 1 Tbs. butter. Spread on top of everything and chill. This takes a little "fussing", but is absolutely worth the effort!

Luscious Lemon Pots de Crème

Basic Stuff

6 8 oz. ceramic custard cups (ramekins)
6 egg yokes
1½ c. heavy cream
½ c. fresh lemon juice
½ c. sugar

Cooking Directions

Mix the lemon juice and sugar in a small bowl until sugar completely dissolves. Whisk the egg yolks and cream together until smooth. Add lemon/sugar mixture to egg/cream mixture; mix thoroughly. Strain through cheesecloth into ramekins. Place ramekins in baking dish. Add hot water to reach 1/2 way up the sides of the ramekins. Bake in 325° oven for 55 minutes, or until soft in their centers. Remove ramekins from oven and baking dish and cool. Refrigerate for at least 3 hours or overnight. This is a palate-pleasing portion of paradise!

Happy Banana Split

Basic Stuff

¼ lb. melted margarine
4 or 5 bananas
1 large can crushed pineapple, drained
2 eggs
1 8 oz. container of Cool Whip
2 c. graham cracker crumbs
½ c. (2 sticks) soft margarine
2 c. powdered sugar
½ c. chopped walnuts
¼ c. crushed pineapple juice
1 tsp. vanilla
1 tsp. cinnamon

Cooking Directions

Mix crust ingredients and pat into a 9" x 13" pan. Mix the filling ingredients for 15 minutes; pour over crust. Slice bananas lengthwise and soak in pineapple juice. Place on filling. Top with crushed pineapple, Cool Whip and chopped walnuts. The only thing missing is the ice cream!

Carrot-Pineapple Cake

Basic Stuff

1½ c. canola oil
1 small can crushed pineapple, drained
3 eggs
2½ c. flour
2 c. sugar
2 c. grated carrots
1 c. chopped walnuts
1 tsp. baking soda
1 tsp. Kosher or Sea salt
1 tsp. vanilla
1 tsp. cinnamon

Cooking Directions

Cream first three ingredients. Add all the rest and mix well.
Bake in a greased 9" x 13" pan for 45 minutes at 350°.
This is mouth-watering when topped with a cream cheese
frosting (well, it's mouth-watering anyway, but the frosting
is a bonus!)

Super Simple Snicker Salad

Basic Stuff

5-6 large Snickers bars, frozen
4-5 Granny Smith apples, unpeeled and chopped
1 12-oz. container Cool-Whip
1 can diced pineapple, drained (optional)

Cooking Directions

Unwrap candy bars and wrap them in a clean cloth. Grab a medium hammer and smack 'em hard into medium pieces. Mix candy and Cool Whip, chopped apples and pineapple if desired. How simple is that? Very tasty stuff!

Succulent Strawberry-Rhubarb Delight

Basic Stuff

2 pints strawberries
3 c. chopped rhubarb
1 c. sugar
¾ c. oatmeal
¾ c. flour
¾ c. sugar
6 Tbs. softened butter
1 Tbs. cornstarch
1 tsp. nutmeg
½ tsp. Kosher or Sea salt

Cooking Directions

Mix the topping ingredients on low speed. Mix the filling ingredients well and pour into a square baking dish. Add topping and bake at 400° for 40 minutes. Great topped with whipping cream or served with ice cream.

Brenda's Blessed Berry Bars

Basic Stuff

4 eggs
1 can strawberry pie filling
8 oz. of cream cheese
3 c. flour
2 c. powdered sugar
1¾ c. sugar
1 c. margarine
2 Tbs. heavy cream
1½ tsp. baking powder
1 tsp. vanilla extract
½ tsp. salt

Cooking Directions

Cream margarine, sugar and 4 oz. of the cream cheese. Add the egg and the vanilla and mix in. Add the flour baking powder and salt. Beat mixture until fully blended. Save approximately 1½ cups of the batter and set aside. Spread the remaining batter onto a greased and floured 15" x 18" jelly roll pan. Spread the strawberry pie filling over the batter. Top the strawberry filling with the saved 1½ cups batter. Bake at 350° for 20 to 25 minutes. While baking, make a glaze by combining 2 cups of powdered sugar, 4 oz. cream cheese and the heavy cream. After baking, let cool and apply glaze mixture. Enjoy this berry-delightful fruity concoction with your best friends after a fine poultry meal.

Iowa Peanut Butter Swirls

Basic Stuff

2 eggs, beaten
1¾ c. milk chocolate morsels
1 c. flour
¾ c. sugar
¾ c. brown sugar packed
½ c. peanut butter
¼ c. butter
2 tsp. vanilla extract
1½ tsp. baking powder
¼ tsp. salt
¼ tsp. Amaretto

Cooking Directions

Pre-heat oven to 350°. Grease a 13" x 9" x 2" baking pan
and set aside. In a bowl, combine the flour, baking powder
and salt. In a medium saucepan cook and stir peanut
butter and butter over low heat until melted. Stir in sugar
and brown sugar. Remove from heat. Stir in eggs and
vanilla. Stir in flour mixture. Spread out in prepared pan.
Sprinkle the morsels on top. Bake 5 minutes then using a
knife, swirl the melted morsels into the rest of the mixture.
Bake about 25 minutes or unitl inserted toothpick comes
out clean. Cool and cut into bars.

Index

Notes and Creative Musings

Notes and Creative
Musings

Notes and Creative Musings

Cary Black lives in Michigan with his family. In his real job, Cary is an R&D Manager for a major Michigan manufacturing company. He has worked as a geologist, researcher, analytical chemist, freelance technical writer, materials scientist, and quality engineer. He is active in the Society of Plastic Engineers, ASTM, and the American Society for Quality.

A native of the Pacific Northwest, Cary spends his free time practicing martial arts, enjoying his children, playing music in the rock band "No Regrets", cooking chicken, and dabbling in the publishing industry with his company, Red Owl Publications.

Don Black lives in Washington State. Since retiring from sales, Don enjoys his time driving a school bus, playing his trombone, and drawing chicken cartoons and other illustrations as a freelance cartoonist.